Immunomodulators and Biologics in Dermatologic Treatment

Neal Bhatia
Editor

Immunomodulators and Biologics in Dermatologic Treatment

Turning Theory into Practice

Springer

Editor
Neal Bhatia
Therapeutics Clinical Research
San Diego, CA, USA

ISBN 978-3-031-66589-9 ISBN 978-3-031-66590-5 (eBook)
https://doi.org/10.1007/978-3-031-66590-5

This Springer imprint is published by the registered company Springer Nature Switzerland AG
The registered company address is: Gewerbestrasse 11, 6330 Cham, Switzerland

Contents

Introduction

Neal Bhatia, Nicole Naterelli, and Nimrit Gahoonia

Abstract The immune system's influence on the skin knows no bounds. The impact on the barrier, the microbiome, the ability to heal wounds, and the manifestations of disease among other consequences are commonly the result of immune dysfunction or immunosuppression. In addition, the range of immunological influences from cellular and humoral immunity can be characterized by many clinical signs and symptoms. The modification of immune processes by therapeutic intervention is meant to modify a disease and, in a sense, "turn off the faucet" that makes a disease rather than simply "mop up the mess" of inflammation that is often a temporary bandage. The individual chapters of this book will review and discuss pathogenesis of diseases and immune mechanisms influencing the skin, as well as multiple topical and systemic approaches to immunomodulation that will match the mechanisms of diseases to the mechanisms of action of therapies.

Keywords Immune · Inhibition · Kinase · Phosphodiesterase · Suppression

1 Immunomodulation

Diseases such as atopic dermatitis, psoriasis, and other dermatoses that originate from Th1, Th2, or Th17 dysfunctions require modulation of the processes that propagate the rashes which were once only treated with steroids. By contrast, immunomodulators represent a unique pharmacologic class of small molecules or substances that indirectly target a disease or pathogen via modulation of the endogenous immune

N. Bhatia (✉)
Therapeutics Clinical Research, San Diego, CA, USA
e-mail: bhatiaharbor@gmail.com

N. Naterelli
Morsani College of Medicine, University of South Florida, 560 Channelside Drive, Tampa, FL 33602, USA

N. Gahoonia
Touro University College of Osteopathic Medicine, 1310 Club Dr, Vallejo, CA 94592, USA

N. Bhatia (ed.), *Immunomodulators and Biologics in Dermatologic Treatment*,
https://doi.org/10.1007/978-3-031-66590-5_1

system [1]. There is a vast utility of immunomodulation, as such approaches can be incorporated into treatment regimens for cancer, infections, and a variety of diseases. Immunomodulators include Janus Kinase (JAK) inhibitors, phosphodiesterase inhibitors, immune checkpoint inhibitors (ICIs), and biologics. In addition, integrative, herbal medicines can have immunomodulatory effects [2].

1.1 Small Molecule Inhibitors

2 Janus Kinase Inhibitors

Janus Kinases (JAKs) are multidomain non-receptor tyrosine kinases that function in cellular signal transduction [3]. Together with signal transducers and activators of transcription (STATs), they transfer cellular signals from membrane receptors to the nucleus. In mammals, the JAK/STAT pathway is the primary signaling mechanism for a range of cytokines and growth factors, [4] resulting in the regulation of immunity, inflammation, and hematopoiesis [5]. Upon cytokine stimulation, such as from proinflammatory type II interferon IFN-γ, JAKs phosphorylate STATs, resulting in their dimerization and translocation into the nucleus for transcriptional regulation [3]. Inhibition of this signaling pathway, however, can suppress important cellular signaling implicated in pathological inflammation and disease.

The JAK family most relevant to dermatology consists of four members: JAK1, JAK2, JAK3, and TYK2 [5]. JAK inhibitors are anti-inflammatory molecules that bind one or more enzymatic domains, thus inhibiting STAT phosphorylation and intracellular signaling. Conversely, JAK inhibitors can be selective for one member, such as JAK1. JAK1 signaling transduction is particularly implicated in pruritic dermatitis, allergic rhinitis, asthma, and inflammatory bowel diseases. As such, JAK1 inhibitors have been efficacious in the management of such conditions. In contrast, JAK1/JAK2 combined inhibitors have been utilized for rheumatoid arthritis, psoriasis, and pruritus [5].

JAK inhibitors have been approved for a variety of conditions, including but not limited to rheumatoid arthritis, ulcerative colitis, atopic dermatitis, alopecia areata, myelofibrosis, and polycythemia vera. Table 1 lists approved JAK inhibitors and their associated uses. In addition, researchers and clinicians have assessed the efficacy of JAK inhibitors for use in the treatment of vitiligo [6, 7]. There is great interest in anti-inflammatory alternatives to the use of topical or oral steroids, which are associated with a multitude of side effects and risks.

Side effects of JAK inhibitors may include but are not limited to headache, cough, dizziness, fatigue, nausea, shortness of breath, and bowel disturbances. In addition, a variety of adverse events have been reported with use. A retrospective review of 126,815 reports from the World Health Organization pharmacovigilance database identified adverse events associated with the first three approved JAK inhibitors: ruxolitinib, tofacitinib, and baricitinib [8]. All three JAK inhibitors were associated

Table 1 JAK inhibitors and their approved uses

Name	Inhibition	Approved uses
Abrocitinib	JAK1	Atopic Dermatitis
Baricitinib	JAK1/JAK2	COVID-19, Rheumatoid Arthritis, Alopecia Areata
Ruxolitinib	JAK1/JAK2	Atopic Dermatitis (topical), Chronic Graft versus Host Disease, Myelofibrosis, Non-Segmental Vitiligo (topical), Polycythemia Vera
Tofacitinib	JAK1/JAK2/JAK3	Ankylosing Spondylitis, Polyarticular Course Juvenile Idiopathic Arthritis, Psoriatic Arthritis, Rheumatoid Arthritis, Ulcerative Colitis
Upadacitinib	JAK1/JAK2	Atopic Dermatitis, Ankylosing Spondylitis, Axial spondyloarthritis, Psoriatic Arthritis, Rheumatoid Arthritis, Ulcerative Colitis

with infectious adverse events, including viral, fungal, and mycobacterial infections, musculoskeletal and connective tissue disorders, embolism and thrombosis, and neoplasms, especially of the skin. Furthermore, tofacitinib was associated with gastrointestinal perforation events [8].

The COMFORT trials, assessing the safety and efficacy of ruxolitinib, found ecchymosis, headache, dizziness, abdominal pain, fatigue, and diarrhea to be the most common nonhematologic adverse events reported [9]. Anemia and thrombocytopenia were the most common hematological adverse events due to JAK2 inhibition, which functions in erythropoietin and thrombopoietin signaling. Lastly, higher rates of herpes zoster infection and basal cell and squamous cell carcinomas have been reported among patients taking ruxolitinib [9].

On September 1, 2021, the Food and Drug Administration (FDA) announced revisions to the black box warnings for JAK inhibitors based on results from the ORAL surveillance study [10]. The randomized controlled study compared treatment outcomes among patients with rheumatoid arthritis with two experimental treatment arms (oral tofacitinib 5 or 10 mg daily) and two comparative arms (40 mg subcutaneous adalimumab injection biweekly or 50 mg subcutaneous etanercept injection weekly, both tumor necrosis factor (TNF) inhibitors). The revised black box warning includes risk information regarding serious cardiac events, malignancy, thrombosis, and death. Although JAK inhibitors have been shown to be efficacious for a variety of inflammatory disorders, their use is associated with a multitude of important risks. While the more selective JAK inhibitors do not appear to carry the same risk and side effect profile, they still carry the black box warning that will require careful discussion with the patient.

Table 2 PDE4 inhibitors and their approved uses

Name	Approved uses
Apremilast	Plaque Psoriasis, Psoriatic Arthritis, Oral Ulcers (Behçet's Disease)
Crisaborole	Atopic Dermatitis (Topical)
Roflumilast	Chronic Obstructive Pulmonary Disease, Psoriasis (Topical), Atopic Dermatitis (pending), Seborrheic Dermatitis (pending)

3 Phosphodiesterase-4 Inhibitors

Phosphodiesterase-4 (PDE4) is a major intracellular non-receptor enzyme class that regulates systemic inflammation. PDE4 hydrolyzes cyclic adenosine monophosphate (cAMP), an important intracellular second messenger that controls proinflammatory and anti-inflammatory mediators [11]. A variety of hematopoietic cells are affected by PDE4 and cAMP concentrations, such as dendritic cells, T cells, macrophages, and monocytes. In addition, keratinocytes, smooth muscle, vascular endothelium, and chondrocytes are mesenchymal cells expressing PDE4 [11].

PDE4 inhibitors block the enzymatic hydrolysis of cAMP, resulting in elevated cAMP concentrations with resulting downstream effects. In lay terms, PDE4 inhibitors function to reduce inflammation mediating a variety of inflammatory pulmonary, dermatological, and neurological diseases [12]. For example, Apremilast, an oral PDE4 inhibitor approved for the treatment of psoriatic arthritis and Behçet's disease, has been shown to decrease interferon-α production and T-cell cytokine production, albeit with little effect on B-cell immunoglobulin secretion [13]. Table 2 lists approved PDE4 inhibitors and their associated uses.

3.1 *Safety*

The most commonly reported adverse effects of oral PDE4 inhibitors have included nausea, vomiting, diarrhea, abdominal pain, weight loss, headache, nasopharyngitis, and upper respiratory tract infections [14]. Apremilast has been associated with development of depression and is also contraindicated in pregnancy [12]. Additionally, Crisaborole has been associated with application site stinging and burning [15].

4 Biologics

Biologics are a class of drugs composed of substances made from living organisms or their products, such as genes, antibodies, receptors, enzymes, inhibitors, and other proteins [16]. Often produced via recombinant DNA technology, biologics are used to manage a variety of inflammatory diseases, in addition to malignancies such as

HER2-positive breast cancer. Immunomodulating biologics are used in the management of rheumatoid arthritis, ankylosing spondylitis, psoriasis, inflammatory bowel disease, and multiple sclerosis [16].

As a diverse class of medication, biologics can regulate inflammation via a variety of mechanisms. Some biologics prevent pro-inflammatory cytokines from binding with extracellular receptors, thereby inhibiting downstream cellular signaling implicated in the pathophysiology of inflammatory disease. Biologics can bind directly with the receptor or neutralize pro-inflammatory cytokines with antibodies [17]. In addition, recombinant anti-inflammatory cytokines can be introduced.

Common targets for biologics used within dermatology include TNF, immune cells such as B and T cells, and cytokines such as IL-1, IL-6, IL-12, IL-17, and IL-23. Biologics are used in the treatment of a wide array of diseases, including Crohn's disease, ulcerative colitis, psoriatic arthritis, psoriasis, rheumatoid arthritis, juvenile idiopathic arthritis, giant cell arteritis, ankylosing spondylitis, and lupus. Table 3 lists biologics commonly used today.

Many of the adverse effects noted from the use of biologics can be explained by their direct suppression of the immune system. These side effects include serious infections from opportunistic pathogens, and tuberculosis reactivation infections.

Table 3 Common biologics and their approved uses

Biologic category	Examples	Approved uses
TNF inhibitor	Adalimumab	Crohn's Disease, Hidradenitis Suppurativa, Juvenile Idiopathic Arthritis, Psoriasis, Psoriatic Arthritis, Rheumatoid Arthritis, Ulcerative Colitis, Uveitis
	Etanercept	Ankylosing Spondylitis, Juvenile Idiopathic Arthritis, Plaque Psoriasis, Psoriatic Arthritis, Rheumatoid Arthritis
	Infliximab	Ankylosing Spondylitis, Crohn's Disease, Psoriasis, Psoriatic Arthritis, Rheumatoid Arthritis, Ulcerative Colitis
IL-17 inhibitor	Brodalumab	Plaque Psoriasis
	Ixekizumab	Ankylosing Spondylitis, Plaque Psoriasis, Psoriatic Arthritis
	Secukinumab	Ankylosing Spondylitis, Enthesitis-Related Arthritis, Non-Radiographic Axial Spondyloarthritis, Plaque Psoriasis, Psoriatic Arthritis
IL-23 inhibitor	Guselkumab	Plaque Psoriasis, Psoriatic Arthritis
	Risankizumab	Crohn's Disease, Plaque Psoriasis, Psoriatic Arthritis
	Tildrakizumab	Plaque Psoriasis
IL-4 and IL-13 inhibitor	Dupilumab	Asthma, Atopic Dermatitis, Chronic Rhinosinusitis with Nasal Polyps, Eosinophilic Esophagitis, Prurigo Nodularis
IL-13 inhibitor	Tralokinumab	Atopic Dermatitis
IL-13 inhibitor	Lebrikizumab	Atopic Dermatitis

Tocilizumab has been especially noted to alter lipid profiles [18]. Rituximab has also shown to cause HBV reactivation and rashes [19]. Additionally, many of the biologics have been associated with causing injection site reactions and infusion reactions [20].

References

1. Nijnik A. Immunomodulatory approaches for prevention and treatment of infectious diseases. Curr Opin Microbiol. 2013;16(5):590–5. https://doi.org/10.1016/j.mib.2013.06.011.
2. Immunomodulators Inspired by Nature: A Review on Curcumin and Echinacea—PubMed. https://pubmed-ncbi-nlm-nih-gov.ezproxy.lib.usf.edu/30373170/. Accessed 15 Dec 2022.
3. McLornan DP, Pope JE, Gotlib J, Harrison CN. Current and future status of JAK inhibitors. Lancet. 2021;398(10302):803–16. https://doi.org/10.1016/S0140-6736(21)00438-4.
4. Rawlings JS, Rosler KM, Harrison DA. The JAK/STAT signaling pathway. J Cell Sci. 2004;117(Pt 8):1281–3. https://doi.org/10.1242/jcs.00963.
5. Shawky AM, Almalki FA, Abdalla AN, Abdelazeem AH, Gouda AM. A comprehensive overview of globally approved JAK inhibitors. Pharmaceutics. 2022;14(5):1001. https://doi.org/10.3390/pharmaceutics14051001.
6. Liu LY, Strassner JP, Refat MA, Harris JE, King BA. Repigmentation in vitiligo using the Janus kinase inhibitor tofacitinib may require concomitant light exposure. J Am Acad Dermatol. 2017;77(4):675-682.e1. https://doi.org/10.1016/j.jaad.2017.05.043.
7. Komnitski M, Komnitski A, Komnitski Junior A, Silva de Castro CC. Partial repigmentation of vitiligo with tofacitinib, without exposure to ultraviolet radiation. An Bras Dermatol. 2020;95(4):473–6. https://doi.org/10.1016/j.abd.2019.08.032.
8. Hoisnard L, Lebrun-Vignes B, Maury S, et al. Adverse events associated with JAK inhibitors in 126,815 reports from the WHO pharmacovigilance database. Sci Rep. 2022;12(1):7140. https://doi.org/10.1038/s41598-022-10777-w.
9. Haq M, Adnan G. Ruxolitinib. In: StatPearls. StatPearls Publishing; 2022. http://www.ncbi.nlm.nih.gov/books/NBK570600/. Accessed 16 Dec 2022.
10. Waiting for JAK inhibitor safety data—PubMed. https://pubmed-ncbi-nlm-nih-gov.ezproxy.lib.usf.edu/35197363/. Accessed 16 Dec 2022.
11. Ilowite NT, Laxer RM. Chapter 13—Pharmacology: biologics. In: Petty RE, Laxer RM, Lindsley CB, Wedderburn LR, editors. Textbook of pediatric rheumatology, Seventh ed. W.B. Saunders; 2016. p. 161–175.e6. https://doi.org/10.1016/B978-0-323-24145-8.00013-2.
12. Li H, Zuo J, Tang W. Phosphodiesterase-4 inhibitors for the treatment of inflammatory diseases. Front Pharmacol. 2018;9:1048. https://doi.org/10.3389/fphar.2018.01048.
13. Schafer PH, Parton A, Capone L, et al. Apremilast is a selective PDE4 inhibitor with regulatory effects on innate immunity. Cellular Signaling. 2014;26(9):2016–29. https://doi.org/10.1016/j.cellsig.2014.05.014.
14. Crocetti L, Floresta G, Cilibrizzi A, Giovannoni MP. An overview of PDE4 inhibitors in clinical trials: 2010 to early 2022. Molecules. 2022;27(15):4964. https://doi.org/10.3390/molecules27154964.
15. Geng B, Hebert AA, Takiya L, et al. Efficacy and safety trends with continuous, long-term crisaborole use in patients aged $\geq$ 2 years with mild-to-moderate atopic dermatitis. Dermatol Ther (Heidelb). 2021;11(5):1667–78. https://doi.org/10.1007/s13555-021-00584-y.
16. Starr SP. Immunology update: biologics. FP Essent. 2016;450:11–21.
17. Rider P, Carmi Y, Cohen I. Biologics for targeting inflammatory cytokines, clinical uses, and limitations. Int J Cell Biol. 2016;2016:9259646. https://doi.org/10.1155/2016/9259646.
18. Souto A, Salgado E, Maneiro JR, Mera A, Carmona L, Gómez-Reino JJ. Lipid profile changes in patients with chronic inflammatory arthritis treated with biologic agents and Tofacitinib

in randomized clinical trials: a systematic review and meta-analysis. Arthritis Rheumatology. 2015;67(1):117–27. https://doi.org/10.1002/art.38894.
19. Kasi PM, Tawbi HA, Oddis CV, Kulkarni HS. Clinical review: serious adverse events associated with the use of rituximab—a critical care perspective. Crit Care. 2012;16(4):231. https://doi.org/10.1186/cc11304.
20. Singh JA, Wells GA, Christensen R, et al. Adverse effects of biologics: a network meta-analysis and Cochrane overview. Cochrane Database Syst Rev. 2011;2011(2):CD008794. https://doi.org/10.1002/14651858.CD008794.pub2.
21. Brzostek J, Gascoigne NRJ, Rybakin V. Cell type-specific regulation of immunological synapse dynamics by B7 ligand recognition. Front Immunol. 2016;7:24. https://doi.org/10.3389/fimmu.2016.00024.
22. Morgado M, Plácido A, Morgado S, Roque F. Management of the adverse effects of immune checkpoint inhibitors. Vaccines (Basel). 2020;8(4):575. https://doi.org/10.3390/vaccines8040575.

Mechanism of Action of Immunomodulators in Dermatologic Disease

Immunomodulators and Dermatology

Sheiva Fakhraie, Caroline Mann, and Raj Chovatiya

Abstract Fundamental knowledge of the mechanisms of action of therapies is necessary to fully understand the immunopathogenesis of dermatologic disease. In recent years, broadly-acting conventional immunosuppressive therapies have given way to safer, more targeted biologic and small molecule therapies that directly target relevant disease-specific pathways. This chapter summarizes the old, new, and future mechanisms of action of immunomodulators and their potential applications to immune-mediated dermatologic disease.

Keywords Immunomodulator · Inflammation · Immunology · Dermatology · Biologic · JAK

1 Introduction

The human body is under constant threat from a wide variety of challenges that can disrupt homeostasis. While this classically includes ancient threats such as microbial pathogens (i.e., bacteria, viruses, and fungi) or multicellular parasites, it can more broadly include environmental allergens, toxins, irritants, and proteases, alongside intrinsic challenges such as metabolic stress, oxidative stress, or even malignant transformation. Over millions of years, the immune system and inflammatory

S. Fakhraie
Department of Dermatology, Northwestern University Feinberg School of Medicine, Chicago, USA

C. Mann
Department of Dermatology, Johannes Gutenberg University Hospital, Mainz, Germany

R. Chovatiya (✉)
Chicago Medical School, Rosalind Franklin University of Medicine and Science, North Chicago, USA
e-mail: raj.chovatiya@rosalindfranklin.edu

Center for Medical Dermatology + Immunology Research, Chicago, USA

N. Bhatia (ed.), *Immunomodulators and Biologics in Dermatologic Treatment*,
https://doi.org/10.1007/978-3-031-66590-5_2

response has evolved to provide protection to a wide variety of potential insults. The immune system constitutes a network of physical, chemical, cellular, and microbiologic barriers designed to detect and respond to a broad array of challenges [1]. In particular, the immune system has the capability to detect a wide array of potential antigens due to specialized cells of the hematopoietic system. These cells have the ability to communicate with each other, as well as other non-immune cells to eliminate and develop lasting memory in order to enhance future immune responses and regulate the response as to not be too strong. Recognizing these important interactions can help us understand the diverse disease states that occur when these interactions are dysregulated, and in turn, understand how targeted therapeutics can treat the many different manifestations of immune-mediated inflammatory disease.

Immune dysregulation plays a key role in many skin diseases. Not only does the skin provide a physical barrier to pathogen entry, but it also contains resident immune and non-immune cells that maintain homeostasis, defend, and repair damaged tissue. Numerous disease states can be thought of as inappropriate (i.e., over- or underactive) immune responses in the skin. This chapter is designed to provide an overview of the cutaneous immune system and provide perspective about the myriad therapeutics used to target different aspects of immunologic disease. Herein, we discuss basic concepts of immunology including types of immunity, roles of hematopoietic cell lineages, and individual cell types, while highlighting the role of skin in the immune system. We will then discuss relevant therapeutic targets by previewing the many immunomodulators used in treatment of dermatologic disease that will be highlighted in the remainder of this book. This chapter is not intended to be a comprehensive review of cutaneous immunology or treatment, but rather, functions as an introduction to basic immunology concepts and major immune modules as they relate to skin pathology in the context of immune dysregulation. In doing so, we hope to build a foundation to better understand immunomodulators in treating skin disease.

2 Basic Concepts of the Immune System

2.1 Types of Immunity

Our immune system is divided into two major programs of immunity: innate immunity and adaptive immunity. The innate immune system is the body's first line of defense against invading pathogens working on a scale of minutes to hours [2]. This form of immunity utilizes the broad concept of pattern recognition to respond to a wide variety of potential insults, and is thus incapable of forming immunologic memory in the event of re-exposure to the same antigen. The adaptive immune system differs in that it is antigen specific, i.e., only responds to specific antigens. As a result, this type of immunity takes much longer from time of exposure to effect, working on a scale of days to weeks [2]. A key feature of adaptive immunity is immunologic memory, the ability to recognize a previously encountered antigen and mount a faster, targeted, and efficient immunologic response. The innate and adaptive immune system do not function in isolation of one other, but rather as simultaneously active, complementary systems.

2.2 *Innate Immunity*

The innate immune system can be thought of possessing several key barriers: physical, physiologic, phagocytic/endocytic, and inflammatory. Physical barriers include the skin and mucous membranes (e.g., pulmonary epithelium). Both the skin and mucous membranes have resident flora that compete with other microbes for attachment sites. In the case of the skin, the pH of the skin is low (4.1–5.8) [3] making it inhospitable for many microbes. The innate immune system is also responsible for systemic physiological changes such as elevations in core body temperature—inhibiting growth of some microorganisms. Cells of the innate immune system use endocytosis or phagocytosis to break down foreign molecules and organisms for elimination from the body. Lastly, tissue damage from invading pathogens induces an inflammatory response in which vascular fluid leaks from vessels bringing with it inflammatory cells and antimicrobial serum proteins.

The innate immune system utilizes pattern recognition receptors (PRRs) to identify a wide variety of pathogens that share similar structural elements known as pathogen associated molecular patterns (PAMPs). There are 3 types of PRRs: the secreted type functions as an opsonin, flagging pathogens for phagocytosis; the endocytic type exist on the surface of phagocytes and facilitate endocytosis; and the signaling type activate intracellular signaling pathways directly.

Activation of the innate immune response leads to the production of cytokines, interferons, and a variety of other mediators that transmit signals to both immune and non-immune cells and activate the inflammatory cascade. Key cytokines in the acute phase of the inflammatory response include tumor necrosis factor alpha (TNFα) and interleukins 1 and 6 (IL-1, IL-6) [4]. Among their many functions, these signals are responsible for priming the activation of the adaptive immune response (which can only be activated after initial recognition by the innate immune system). Many inflammatory and autoimmune diseases can occur as a result of these cytokines, making them important targets for treatments. Cells of the innate immune system include granulocytes (neutrophils, basophils, and eosinophils), macrophages, dendritic cells, mast cells, natural killer cells, and innate lymphoid cells.

2.3 *Adaptive Immunity*

In contrast to the innate immune system, the adaptive immune system continues to develop with age and exposure to environmental antigens. The adaptive immune systems functions to more specifically identify "self" from "non-self," generate a targeted response to a particular antigen, and develop immunologic memory to protect from subsequent exposure. The main cells of the adaptive immune system include T and B lymphocytes. During development, the genes encoding the receptors for these cells undergo a process of V(D)J recombination which is critical in creating an incredibly diverse population of B and T cell receptors that are capable of detecting any potential pathogenic antigen [5]. Thus, each lymphocyte contains a unique receptor capable of recognizing only a single antigen. During the process of V(D)J recombination, receptors recognizing self-antigen can also be produced; however, these cells are targeted for elimination early in their maturation process. When mature lymphocytes recognize their specific antigen, clonal proliferation is stimulated with the help of antigen presenting cells (APCs) of the innate immune system.

T and B lymphocytes develop from common lymphoid progenitor cells that develop in the bone marrow. T lymphocytes then mature in the thymus and B lymphocytes mature in the bone marrow. B and T lymphocytes then migrate to the secondary lymphoid organs the lymph nodes and spleen where they reside until activation. Once activated, lymphocytes can emerge from these secondary lymphoid organs and migrate to sites of infection through the effects of cellular adhesion molecules and chemokine receptors. Upon initial encounter with an antigen, a set of long-lived memory B and T cells develop for more rapid and robust response upon future chalet [6].

APCs display antigens on one of two types of major histocompatibility complexes (MHC I and MHC II). There are three major classes of T cells: T helper cells (CD4+ T cells), cytotoxic T cells (CD8+ T cells), and regulatory T cells. Cytotoxic T cells contain a CD8 receptor that is capable of recognizing antigens presented on MHC class I molecules. MHC class 1 molecules are found on both APCs as well as all other nucleated cells in the human body—allowing for direct elimination of infected or altered cells. CD4+ ("helper") T cells possess a CD4 receptor that recognizes antigens on MHC class II molecules, which are found exclusively on APCs. The main role of these T cells is to modify the activity of other immune cells through the release of cytokines and other mediators. Regulatory T cells modulate the immune response by suppressing activity of various aspects of the immune response.

Unlike T cells, B-cell receptors can identify an antigen directly—i.e., an antigen does not have to be present on an MHC molecule for detection. Thus, B cells can undergo T-cell independent and dependent forms of activation. When B cells become activated, they turn into antibody producing plasma cells. Antibodies function to neutralize infectivity, aid in phagocytosis, assist in antibody dependent cellular cytotoxicity, and facilitate complement mediated lysis of pathogens or infected cells [7].

2.4 *The Skin's Role in the Immune System*

The skin is a large, complex organ that plays an important role in our immune system. The skin has physical, chemical, and microbiological barriers to entry for invading microbes. This role is critical for the maintenance of tissue homeostasis, defense, and repair in the case of tissue injury. The skin contains an intricate network of skin structures, resident, and non-resident immune cells that all work together to accomplish this defense. The epidermis, the outermost layer of our skin, plays both a passive and active role in the defense from the external environment. Keratinocytes in the epidermis provide physical protection from microbes, UV light, chemical and physical stress.

The outermost layer of the skin, the stratum corneum, is responsible for much of the barrier function of the skin. Corneocytes in the stratum corneum contain lipid envelopes anchored to keratin filaments increasing the rigidity of the barrier [8]. The barrier function of the skin is also largely dependent on adhesion molecules and tight junctions which if impaired, can lead to inflammatory skin conditions [9].

In addition to the physical barrier provided by corneocytes, antimicrobial peptides (AMPs) are important in skin defense mechanisms. AMPs have both an antimicrobial and an immunomodulatory role in the skin's defense [10]. These peptides have been shown to impact immune cell proliferation, migration, and differentiation, to contribute to the skin barrier, and to promote wound healing [11].

The microbiome of the skin also provides a layer of protection against invading pathogens. This microbiome is composed primarily of bacteria, but includes a variety of other commensal species (e.g., Malassezia yeast, demodex mites) that provide a protective layer against colonization with pathogenic microbes. The microenvironment of the skin barrier typically allows only for colonization by certain species, and thus, any physiological change that alters this environment can stimulate immune reactions that may drive different disease states.

The skin maintains a relatively low pH [3], creating a difficult environment for microbes to invade. Contributors to this acidic environment include fatty acids found in the stratum corneum, sweat glands acidic contents produced by the sweat glands, and acidic metabolites of filaggrin, a filament associated protein found in the skin [12–14].

In the event of infection or tissue injury, the skin contains resident immune cells that can rapidly identify infection or damage, signal an inflammatory response, and initiate tissue repair. Many immune cells reside in the skin, including Langerhans cells (LCs) and dermal dendritic cells (dDCs), macrophages/monocytes, mast cells, eosinophils, and lymphocytes. Non-immune cells such as keratinocytes and fibroblasts also contribute to the skin's defense and tissue repair.

LCs and dDCs are found in the epidermis and papillary dermis, respectfully, where they are continuously sampling environmental antigens and migrate to regional lymph nodes to either induce tolerance to self-antigens or to mount an adaptive response in the case of non-self-antigens [15]. These cells are professional APCs capable of activating both helper and cytotoxic T cells. In the case of tissue repair, these cells have been found to accelerate early wound healing events [16].

Macrophages in the skin are found in both the papillary and reticular dermis where they have diverse functions in phagocytosis of pathogens, elimination of cellular debris, tissue homeostasis, inflammation, and tissue repair [17]. Macrophages can further be subclassified based on their specialized functions. For example, classical pro-inflammatory macrophages secrete acute phase inflammatory cytokines such as TNFα, IL-1, and IL-6, along with chemokines, to recruit peripheral inflammatory cells and signal inflammation. In contrast, anti-inflammatory macrophages specialized in tissue repair secrete TBFβ and are pro-fibrotic through stimulation of angiogenesis, fibroblast proliferation, collagen synthesis and matrix remodeling [18].

Mast cells, also found in the papillary and reticular dermis, contain pre-formed granules containing histamine, sulfated proteoglycans, serotonin, and tryptase or chymase [19]. Mast cells contain Fcε receptors that bind immunoglobin E (IgE). When mast cells encounter an allergen, the allergen cross links IgE on the mast cell surface releasing the contents of the pre-formed granules. Mast cells also produce large quantities of eicosanoids (e.g., prostaglandins, leukotrienes), another important class of inflammatory mediator.

Eosinophils are found in the reticular dermis and contain granules of major basic protein (MBP), eosinophil peroxidase (EPO) and eosinophil cationic protein (ECP) [20]. In response to eosinophil activation, these granules are released in a pulsatile manner. The differentiation, activation, and degranulation of eosinophils is largely driven by IL-5 produced by type 2 CD4+ helper T cells, mast cells, and other eosinophils Eosinophils primarily provide defense against multicellular helminths and other parasites, but they also play a broader role defense against other organisms.

2.5 Immunomodulatory Strategies to Treat Skin Disease

The idea of using immunomodulation to treat dermatologic disease is not a new concept. Until recently, broad acting immunosuppressants were one of the few available strategies for treating chronic inflammatory and autoimmune skin diseases. In recent years, there has been a revolution in targeted biologic, oral, and topical therapies designed to maximize efficacy, minimize safety risk, and most importantly, promote patient tolerance and adherence. To best understand the unique role that the immune system plays in dermatologic disease and how theory has been turned into practice, in the next section we review traditional immunomodulatory therapeutic classes used to treat dermatologic diseases and then place a special focus on immune system modules targeted newer types of therapies.

3 Traditional Immunodulatory Strategies

3.1 Glucocorticoids

Glucocorticoids (GCs) belong to the family of corticosteroids, a group of hormones produced by the adrenal gland. Topical (e.g., hydrocortisone), oral (e.g., prednisone), and injectable (e.g., methylprednisolone) corticosteroid formulations are common, broadly-used synthetic analogs used for nearly all inflammatory diseases.

The mechanism of action of GCs, both in systemic and topical formulations, involves their binding to specific intracellular GC receptors (GR), encoded by the NR3C1 gene, expressed in various tissues in a cell- and tissue-specific manner [21].

Due to their high lipid content, GCs enter the cell by diffusion. In the cytosol, they bind to receptors that form a complex with heat shock proteins (Hsp70 and Hsp90). The binding subsequently opens a DNA binding site which allows for direct binding to glucocorticoid response elements (GREs) located on target gene enhancers and promoters upon translocation of the GR complex into the nucleus [22].

The binding of the GR complex to GREs can either activate or repress gene transcription, depending on the specific target gene. The expression of up to 1% of all genes can be regulated by GCs—most often upregulation—showing how truly broad acting GCs are as treatment for skin disease [21]. Why some target genes are enhanced, while others are suppressed remains unclear. GCs can stimulate transcription of anti-inflammatory genes, such as cytokine inhibitors, while simultaneously inhibit the transcription of pro-inflammatory genes, such as cytokines and prostaglandins, and induce apoptosis in leukocytes and lymphocytes (Table 1) [23]. By blocking the expression of adhesion molecules, the migration of inflammatory cells into the tissue is further prevented [21, 24].

The effects of GCs on gene expression are wide-ranging and complex, resulting in both beneficial and detrimental effects on the body. For example, GCs can reduce inflammation, suppress the immune system, and regulate metabolism, but they can also cause osteoporosis, weight gain, and mood disturbance [22]. The positive effects of corticosteroids must thus be weighed against the potential negative consequences, particularly those associated with chronic use.

Of particular concern to dermatologists, the effect of topical corticosteroids (TCS) is defined by potency, which is dependent not only the concentration, but also vehicle type and treatment location [23]. In addition to their anti-inflammatory effects at a cellular and molecular level, TCS also exhibit vasoconstrictive properties. This influences the tissue migration of leukocytes but also the number and function of LCs, monocytes, and NK cells in the skin. Another effect, which is beneficial in the treatment of allergic reactions, is the blocking of IgE release from mast cells [23].

3.2 Calcineurin Inhibitors

Cyclosporine (CsA) is a small, cyclic, amino-acid based molecule initially used for prevention of organ transplant rejection and later for the treatment of autoimmune and inflammatory diseases in both oral and injectable formulations. It is also a founding member of the family of calcineurin inhibitors. Calcineurin is a serine/threonine phosphatase, which is activated by increase in cytosolic calcium following activation of T lymphocytes, which leads to dephosphorylation of nuclear factor of activated T-cells (NFAT-1) in the cytoplasm. The transcription factor NFAT-1 translocates into the nucleus, where it binds to DNA sequences which encode for genes such as IL-2, IL-3, IL-4, and IL-5, CD40 and Fas-ligand.

Upon formation of the CsA/cyclophilin complex, calcineurin is effectively inhibited and unable to be activated by calcium flux. Calcineurin-inhibitors therefore exhibit their effect by broadly reducing T-cell proliferation and subsequent cytokine production, which importantly includes IL-2, a key proliferative signal for T cells [25]. While cyclosporine is more specific than GC-based therapies, it also inhibits most adaptive immune responses indiscriminately. Due to presence of target molecules beyond the T cell compartment, side effects (e.g., renal toxicity) are associated with CsA use—however, T cells are still relatively most sensitive to the effects of calcineurin inhibitors. Furthermore, CsA is metabolized through cytochrome P-450, which makes a drug-drug interaction through competitive interaction possible, which can lead to an elevated serum concentration and higher risk of side effects.

The topical calcineurin inhibitors (TCI) pimecrolimus and tacrolimus were first introduced as an alternative topical anti-inflammatory treatment option [26]. Different from CsA, which binds to cyclophilin, TCI bind the immunophilin FK-binding protein-12 (FKBP-12), also known as FKBP1A. The subsequent downstream blocking of calcineurin phosphatase activity is similar to CsA. Pimecrolimus mainly targets T lymphocytes and mast cells, whereas Tacrolimus interacts with T lymphocytes, mast cells, eosinophils, basophils and LCs [27].

Due to their high binding affinity and low rate of skin absorption (hampered by high molecular weight), systemic adverse reactions are less common with TCI, though concern for possible AEs stems mainly from increased permeability in inflamed skin [27]. TCI do not lead to skin atrophy, as they do not influence fibroblasts or endothelial cells like GCs. However, they can cause local adverse effects of skin burning and irritation [28]. In addition, a boxed warning regarding the risk of increased lymphoma risk was released in 2006, however, this risk has since been relativized following long-term studies [29, 30].

3.3 Methotrexate

Methotrexate (MTX) is a folic acid analogue that inhibits several enzymes including dihydrofolate reductase (DHFR), thymidylate synthetase, as well as glycinamide ribonucleotide transformylase (GARFT) and aminoimidazole carboxamide transformylase (AICARFT). This inhibition results in impaired purine and pyrimidine synthesis, which in turn leads to an inability to synthesize DNA or RNA. This effectively inhibits cellular proliferation, which makes MTX a potent anti-inflammatory drug (given effects on the expanding T cell population) with a broad side effect profile (given potential deleterious effects on any dividing cells). The mechanism of action of low-dose MTX is fundamentally different from the cytostatic effects seen at higher doses. At elevated concentrations, MTX inhibits the enzyme AICAR transformylase which is crucial for the production of adenosine, and thereby limits the adenosine dependent adhesion of granulocytes to endothelial cells.

3.4 Mycophenolate Mofetil

The active metabolite of mycophenolate mofetil (MMF) is mycophenolic acid (MPA), which functions as an inhibitor of inosine monophosphate dehydrogenase (IMPDH). IMPDH can be divided into two isoforms a (type I and II) and is essential in the synthesis of guanosine nucleotides, which is needed for T- and B-lymphocyte survival.

The affinity of MPA to type II is comparably higher than type I, explaining its stronger effect on T-lymphocytes. Furthermore, MPA suppresses the expression of adhesion molecules, thus further affecting immune cell recruitment and inhibits the production of nitric oxide, resulting in reduced tissue damage [31].

3.5 Azathioprine

The active metabolite of azathioprine (AZT) is 6-mercaptopurine, which is a purine-analog, and therefore an antagonist of the purine metabolism which affects DNA and RNA synthesis. This results in the major activities of azathioprine through its non-specific effects on proliferating cells, namely the apoptosis of T and B lymphocytes and subsequent reduction of proinflammatory cytokine and immunoglobulin synthesis [32].

3.6 Dapsone

Beyond its use as an antibiotic drug exhibiting bacteriostatic effects, dapsone is favored in the treatment of diseases with neutrophilic infiltrates, as it affects neutrophil function by inhibiting the myeloperoxidase system. This leads to an overall reduction of neutrophils in inflamed tissue. Furthermore, dapsone reduces the production of reactive oxygen species and interferes with eosinophil peroxidase on mast cells, contributing to its immunomodulatory properties [33].

3.7 Cyclophosphamide

Cyclophosphamide is a cyclic nitrogen-lost derivative that exerts its alkylating and phosphorylating effects after being metabolized in the liver. Upon activation, it leads to alkylation of DNA and RNA and interferes with enzymes of the inner and outer cell membrane, resulting in the inhibition of cell proliferation and rapid protein synthesis (hence its use in inhibiting antibody production in B-cell mediated diseases).

3.8 Chloroquine and Hydroxychloroquine

Chloroquine (CQ) and hydroxychloroquine (HCQ) are well-described antimalarial agents. However, because of their ability to alter signaling pathways and transcriptional activity, leading to inhibition of cytokine production, they are commonly used in several autoimmune skin diseases. CQ and HCQ accumulate an acidic compartments such as lysosomes and inflamed tissue. This ability to broadly penetrate across tissue types is leveraged for treatment—though also comes with the risk of side effects with this medication class. Apart from their immunomodulatory effects, CQ and HCQ can also lead to improvement of hyperglycemia, hyperlipidemia, protection against infection [34].

3.9 Immunoglobulin Therapy

Intravenous Immunoglobulin G (IVIG) is prepared from human plasma used to treat a variety of immunodeficiency, inflammatory, and autoimmune conditions. The exact mechanism of action is still not fully understood, however, among various postulated effects, IVIG can lead to a Fc receptor blockade, thus leading to immune cell impairment, complement inhibition, elimination of autoantigens and autoantibody blocking, inhibition of cytokine synthesis and enhanced corticosteroids sensitivity [35].

3.10 Vitamin D

The vitamin D receptor (VDR) is a nuclear receptor which forms a heterodimer with retinoid X receptor alpha (RXR alpha) after binding of 1, 25(OH) 2D3 (calcitriol), the Vitamin D derivative with highest affinity. The activated VDR complex binds to the vitamin D responsive elements (VDRE) on the DNA, where it induces the synthesis of various proteins such as TRPV6 (transient receptor potential V6, a calcium channel), Calbindin-D9K (responsible for calcium transport in enterocytes) and PMCA1b (plasma membrane Ca2+-ATPase, a calcium ATPase) [36, 37]. The VDR influences proliferation and differentiation in a variety of different cell types, including immune cells such as monocytes, macrophages, DCS, NK cells and activated T- and B-cells—explaining the immunomodulatory properties of vitamin D derivatives [36]. Calcitriol can also inhibit the transcription of pro-inflammatory cytokines such as TNF-α, IL-6, and IL-12 in monocytes [38] and the production of RANTES and IL-8, thus inhibiting hyperproliferation of epidermal keratinocytes [39]. VDR has been found on tumoral cells, making it a possible therapeutic target in cancer therapy [40].

3.11 Retinoids

Retinoids, a group of vitamin A derivatives, are natural or synthetic molecules with pleiotropic effects on gene expression and regulation, especially cell growth and differentiation. In a target cell, active natural metabolites retinoic acid (RA) and 9-cis-retinoic acid are synthetized from retinol. There are two groups of retinoid nuclear receptors (RNR): the RA receptors (RARs), which bind RA, and the retinoid X receptors (RXRs), which bind 9-cis-retinoic acid. RXR is mainly expressed by keratinocytes and hair follicle cells, whereas RXRD is found in the epidermis [41]. After binding of the ligand, the retinoid-receptor complexes are transported into the nucleus where they bind specific regulatory DNA sequences (retinoid hormone response elements), thereby stimulating the transcription of target genes. These genes tend to have a regulating effect on keratinocyte differentiation and proliferation (e.g., keratins K1 and K10, involucrin, and filaggrin). This implicates that retinoids can be beneficial in diseases with keratinocyte hyper-proliferation.

4 Targeted Immunomodulatory Strategies

4.1 Phosphodiesterase 4

Phosphodiesterase 4 (PDE4) is an enzyme that catalyzes the hydrolysis of cyclic adenosine monophosphate (cAMP) to adenosine monophosphate (AMP). Four subtypes of PDE4 (A, B, C and D) exist. PDE4A. is expressed in nearly all skin cell types, PDE4B is present in blood vessels and immune cells, and PDE4D is expressed in fibroblasts and endothelial cells [42]. When cAMP levels are high, PDE4 activity increases, and cAMP levels are reduced. Conversely, when cAMP levels are low, PDE4 activity decreases, and cAMP levels increase.

Inhibition of PDE4, which can be accomplished both with topical (crisaborole, roflumilast) and oral (apremilast) medications, results in increased cAMP levels, which promotes an anti-inflammatory effect by reducing activity of T cells, NK cells, and DCs in the skin. Beyond this effect, PDE4 inhibitors have been shown to downregulate the plasma levels of cytokines such as TNF-α, IL-17F, IL-17A, and IL-22 [42, 43].

4.2 Aryl Hydrocarbon Receptor (AhR)

The aryl hydrocarbon receptor (AhR) is expressed primarily at barrier surfaces of the body (including the skin) but also in lymphocytes and other immune cells [44, 45]. The "canonical regulation" of AhR involves the binding of a ligand to the AhR, which leads to its transport into the cell nucleus. In the nucleus, the AhR can bind with the AhR nuclear translocator (ARNT) and induce genes of the AhR gene battery designed to regulate homeostasis and control stress pathways, such as cytochrome P450 (CYP) enzymes. The AhR repressor (AhRR) can inhibit the activation of the AhR and exert a negative, counter-regulatory effect. The AhR system can be influenced by acute exposure to toxic substances such as tetrachlorodibenzo-p-dioxin (TCDD) or by chronic inflammation, leading to the alternative binding of the AhR to other signaling proteins ("non-canonical regulation") such as the epidermal growth factor receptor (EGFR), mitogen-activated protein kinases (MAPK), nuclear factor kappa-light-chain-enhancer of activated B-cells (NF-κB), signal transducers and activators of transcription (STATs), or peroxisome proliferator-activated receptors (PPARs) [46]. Many of the beneficial effects of complex historical therapies like coal tar and more recent targeted molecules like tapinarof are better understood to be mediated by modulation of AhR [45], including regulation of inflammation and keratinocyte differentiation, It is thought that a short-term induction of the AhR nuclear translocation through the use these products can lead to skin barrier normalization and therapeutic effect [45–47].

4.3 Cytokines

Cytokines are secreted by a variety of cells and can exert autocrine, paracrine, and endocrine effects. Major cytokine classes include interleukins (IL), interferons (IFN), chemokines, tumor necrosis factors (TNF), and lymphokines, and each of these classes exerts both distinct and overlapping effects as mediators of inflammation by binding to extracellular receptors and causing changes in gene expression within target cells [25]. CD4+ helper T lymphocytes are one major source of cytokines across a variety of dermatologic diseases. Cutaneous skewing of T lymphocytes results in specialized cellular programs to aid in selective production of different groups of effector cytokines in both host defense and pathogenic states. For example, type 1 helper T cells (Th1) are polarized by IL-12 secrete IFNγ and IL-2; Th2 cells are skewed by IL-4 secrete IL-4 IL-5, IL-10, IL-13; and Th17 cells are skewed by IL-6, TGFβ, and IL-23 and produce IL-17A, IL-17F, IL-21, and IL-22. Recent classification suggests grouping these T-cell mediated inflammatory programs into 3 major inflammatory pathways that are characteristic of distinct disease states. Type 1 inflammation is linked to activation of Th1 cells along with type 1 innate lymphoid cells (ILCs) NK cells, and macrophages, while type 2 inflammation is driven by Th2 cells, alongside type 2 ILCs, eosinophils, basophils and mast cells, and type 3 inflammation with Th17 cells, ILC3, Th22 and neutrophils. However, immune activation occurs across multiple dimensions and cytokines form cross-regulatory networks and play an important role in the growth, development, functional differentiation of immune cells as well as epidermal and dermal cells.

Biologic therapies consist of genetically synthesized monoclonal antibodies, fusion protein products, or even recombinant proteins that specifically modulate the function of cytokines or cytokines while limiting broader issues of immunosuppression or toxicity across the immune system and target tissues [25]. A few selective examples of cytokine pathways targeted by biologic therapies will be presented here to understand the potential of biologic therapies, with a more inclusive and detailed discussion to follow in subsequent chapters.

4.3.1 TNFα

TNFα is a key inflammatory cytokine with pleiotropic functions across different immune modules. It is secreted not only by immune cells but also keratinocytes as well in response to a wide variety of infections and other insults [48, 49]. It has well-described roles in the prevention of intracellular viral and bacterial infections as an organizing cytokine in the Th1 immune response. TNFα also assists in stimulating the production of Th17 signature cytokines, including IL-17 and IL-23, in the response to extracellular bacteria and fungi. Targeting of the TNFα pathway was one of the first successful strategies for specific immunomodulation in any disease state and has shown efficacy in a variety of disease states including dermatologic (psoriasis, hidradenitis suppurativa), rheumatologic (rheumatoid arthritis, psoriatic arthritis), and gastroenterological (inflammatory bowel disease).

4.3.2 IL-4 and IL-13

The type I receptor complex binds IL-4 and consists of the IL-4Rα and the common γ-chain (IL-2Rγ) subunits, which are bound intracellularly by Janus kinases 1 and 2 (JAK1/JAK2). The type II receptor complex binds both IL-4 and IL-13 and consists of IL-4Rα and 13Rα1, which are linked intracellularly to tyrosine kinase 2 (TYK2) and JAK1. Both cytokines share overlapping and distinct functions in type 2 inflammation which is at the core of several different dermatologic diseases including atopic dermatitis. IL4 is appears to uniquely be responsible for initial differentiation of Th2 cells, while IL-13 is most important for sustaining the cutaneous inflammatory response in the skin, leading to immune dysregulation, barrier dysfunction, and microbial dysbiosis. Il-13 is found in higher levels than IL-4 in the skin and correlates well with disease activity [50]. Both share overlapping roles in signaling pruritus on cutaneous afferent neurons.

4.3.3 IL-17

IL-17 is produced by activated Th17 cells and acts on various target cells, including immune cells, epithelial cells, and endothelial cells. IL-17 activates transcription factors including nuclear factor kappa B (NF-κB) and activator protein 1 (AP-1) and upregulates the expression of various proinflammatory genes, including cytokines, chemokines, and adhesion molecules. This leads to the activation and recruitment of immune cells, the synthesis of extracellular matrix components, and the promotion of inflammation. IL-17 also plays a role in the development and maintenance of Th17 cells and has been shown to synergize with other cytokines, such as IL-6 and IL-23, to promote Th17 differentiation. In addition, IL-17 has been shown to have both positive and negative regulatory effects on T cell function and to modulate the activity of other immune cells, such as neutrophils, macrophages, and dendritic cells [51, 52]. These functions are especially relevant in psoriatic disease as well as non-dermatologic conditions (e.g., ankylosing spondylitis).

4.3.4 IL-23

IL-23 is a cytokine that plays several roles in inflammation, immune activation, and hyperproliferation of the stratum corneum. IL-23 is a heterodimer consisting of two subunits: p40, which is shared with IL-12 in the Th1 pathway, and p19, which is specific to IL-23. The expression of retinoic acid-related orphan receptors (RORs) can activate the production of IL-23 by antigen-presenting cells (APCs) and myeloid dendritic cells, which then act on the entire Th17 and Th22 axis in psoriatic disease [49, 53].

4.3.5 IL-31

IL-31 is produced predominantly by Th2 cells and stimulates neurons directly to induce itch, and it also negatively influences the expression of filaggrin, thus leading to skin barrier dysfunction [54]. Targeting of IL-31 could thus positively influence multiple aspects of skin biology and is of particular interest in type 2 inflammatory diseases associated with itch, such as atopic dermatitis and prurigo nodularis.

4.3.6 IL-36

IL-36 is a part of the IL-1 family and mainly expressed in the skin. The IL-36 receptor activates dendritic cells and stimulates T-cell polarization. IL-36 is of special relevance in generalized pustular psoriasis, where many cases are associated with a mutation in the IL-36 receptor antagonist protein (IL-36RN), resulting in constant activation of IL-36 and other downstream cytokines like IL-6. Blocking the IL-36 receptor results in reduced activity of NFκB signaling as well as cytokines like IFNɣ, IL-4, IL-17 and IL-22 [55].

4.3.7 IL-1

IL-1 physiologically binds to membrane-bound IL-1 receptor type 1, and the receptor-ligand complex then forms a heterodimeric complex with the accessory protein IL-1RacP. Through this complex, an intracellular signaling cascade is triggered during inflammation. The pathway is often aberrantly activated in autoinflammatory diseases, and thus, the goal of treatment is centered around achieving better balance of IL-1 receptor antagonism. Inhibition of interleukin-1 prevents neutrophil recruitment to joints, macrophage activation, and T and B lymphocyte differentiation, which secondarily reduces bone and cartilage destruction as well as swelling and intra-articular pain.

4.4 IgE

IgE is initially produced by B cells and response to antigen presentation and is responsible for degranulation and histamine release from mast cells and basophils. It plays a central role in the pathogenesis of allergic inflammation. Anti-IgE based therapies neutralize free IgE by binding with both FcεRI and CD23, as well as binding membrane IgE that is part of the B-cell receptor (BCR) [56].

4.5 JAK-STAT Signaling

Janus kinases (JAKs) are intracellular enzymes that play a major role in cytokine signal transduction pathways. They are activated when cytokines bind to a type I or II receptor and lead to phosphorylation of signal transducers and activator of transcription (STATs). The STAT proteins then form dimers by binding phosphotyrosine residues in SH2 pockets and translocate into the nucleus in an importin α-5 dependent manner via the Ran nuclear import pathway, where they then activate the transcription of a variety of genes that play a role in adaptive immunity. Among its many functions, JAK-STAT pathway has a critical role in the fate of T helper cells

(Th) and their differentiation into effector subsets, including Th1, Th2, Th17 and regulatory T cells (Tregs).

JAK inhibitors consist of small molecules that bind to JAKs and block signaling pathways that contribute to inflammation and immune system activation. By inhibiting these pathways selectively yet broadly, JAK inhibitors can target the symptoms of many different autoimmune and inflammatory skin disorders by modulating gene expression, protein synthesis, and cell proliferation [57, 58], including atopic dermatitis, psoriasis, alopecia areata, vitiligo, and connective tissue disease. There are four different members of the Janus kinase family: JAK 1, JAK 2, JAK 3 and TYK2. There are more than 90 different JAK inhibitors available worldwide, however, only a small percentage are in clinical development, in part related to the required specificity for disease immunomodulation [59]. While available medications are generally well-tolerated, they can be associated with increased risk for infection, venous thromboembolism, cardiovascular disease, malignancy, and cytopenias in certain clinical contexts [21, 60].

4.6 *Immunologic Checkpoints*

The increased understanding of the role of the immune system in the treatment of cancer patients led to an understanding of immunologic checkpoints, which are master signals responsible for directing the activity of immune cells. Activation of immune checkpoints are important for tolerance and the resolution phase of immune activity, however, this is often co-opted by malignant cells to create local "immunosuppression" to avoid detection or eradication. Checkpoint inhibitors are designed to overcome immunosuppression induced by the tumor itself and make cancer cells "visible" to the immune system. These checkpoint inhibitors induce a cytotoxic immune response against tumor cells by targeting the transmembrane receptors, which are expressed on the surface of cancer cells and certain immune cells: cytotoxic T lymphocyte-associated protein 4 (CTLA-4), programmed cell death 1 (PD-1), and programmed cell death ligand 1 (PD-L1). PD-1 is transmembrane receptor expressed on the surface of immune cells such as T cells, B cells, NK cells, dendritic cells and monocytes; PD-L1 functions as its ligand and is expressed on the surrounding interacting cells [61]. Normally, when PD-L1 binds to PD-1 on T-cells, it can inhibit the immune response and protect cancer cells from immune cells. The CTLA-4 receptor is expressed on immune cells including myeloid-derived suppressor cells, B cells, and NK cells [62]. CTLA4 belongs to the family of anti-inflammatory immune checkpoints that inhibit the immune reactivity of T lymphocytes and arrest the cell cycle. Currently checkpoint inhibitor therapy is leveraged mainly for the treatment of malignancy, but its principles are in early phases of investigation for immune-mediated inflammatory disease.

5 Conclusion

Dermatology has witnessed a revolution in targeted, immunomodulatory treatment approaches in the past few decades. As we have learned more about the considerable burden of cutaneous and systemic symptoms along with quality-of-life issues associated with chronic immune mediated inflammatory disease, the need to adequately treat our patients with safe and effective options in place of older, broad-acting therapies has never been more pressing. Here we briefly reviewed the basics of immunology for the dermatologist to highlight how theory is finally being put into practice. The next generation of clinicians and investigators will undoubtedly be able to further unravel the complexities of immune dysregulation in skin disease and discover even more innovative treatment approaches than those highlighted here—the future has never looked so bright.

6 Conflicts of Interest

RC has served as an advisor, consultant, speaker, and/or investigator for AbbVie, Amgen, AnaptysBio, Apogee Therapeutics, Arcutis, Argenx, ASLAN Pharmaceuticals, Beiersdorf, Boehringer Ingelheim, Bristol Myers Squibb, Cara Therapeutics, Dermavant, Eli Lilly and Company, FIDE, Formation Bio, Galderma, Genentech, GSK, Incyte, LEO Pharma, L'Oréal, Nektar Therapeutics, Novartis, Opsidio, Pfizer Inc., RAPT, Regeneron, Sanofi, Sitryx, Takeda, TRexBio, and UCB.

SF has no conflicts to disclose.

CM has received personal fees from Almirall, Lilly, Pfizer, and Sanofi.

References

1. Marshall JS, Warrington R, Watson W, Kim HL. An introduction to immunology and immunopathology. Allergy Asthma Clin Immunol. 2018;14(Suppl 2):49.
2. Robertson M. Innate immunity. Curr Biol. 1998;8(17):R595–7.
3. Segger D, Aßmus U, Brock M, Erasmy J, Finkel P, Fitzner A, et al. Multicenter study on measurement of the natural pH of the skin surface. Int J Cosmetic Sci. 2008;30(1):75.
4. Dinarello CA. Proinflammatory cytokines. Chest. 2000;118(2):503–8.
5. Bassing CH, Swat W, Alt FW. The mechanism and regulation of chromosomal V(D)J recombination. Cell. 2002;109(2, Supplement 1):S45–S55.
6. Bonilla FA, Oettgen HC. Adaptive immunity. J Allergy Clin Immunol. 2010;125(2 Suppl 2):S33-40.
7. Forthal DN. Functions of antibodies. Microbiol Spectr. 2014;2(4):1–17.
8. Madison KC. Barrier function of the skin: "la raison d'être" of the epidermis. J Invest Dermatol. 2003;121(2):231–41.
9. Brandner JM, Kief S, Grund C, Rendl M, Houdek P, Kuhn C, et al. Organization and formation of the tight junction system in human epidermis and cultured keratinocytes. Eur J Cell Biol. 2002;81(5):253–63.

10. Niyonsaba F, Kiatsurayanon C, Chieosilapatham P, Ogawa H. Friends or Foes? Host defense (antimicrobial) peptides and proteins in human skin diseases. Exp Dermatol. 2017;26(11):989–98.
11. Herman A, Herman AP. Antimicrobial peptides activity in the skin. Skin Res Technol. 2019;25(2):111–7.
12. Bibel DJ, Miller SJ, Brown BE, Pandey BB, Elias PM, Shinefield HR, et al. Antimicrobial activity of stratum corneum lipids from normal and essential fatty acid-deficient mice. J Invest Dermatol. 1989;92(4):632–8.
13. Krien PM, Kermici M. Evidence for the existence of a self-regulated enzymatic process within the human stratum corneum-an unexpected role for urocanic acid. J Invest Dermatol. 2000;115(3):414–20.
14. Wilke K, Martin A, Terstegen L, Biel SS. A short history of sweat gland biology. Int J Cosmet Sci. 2007;29(3):169–79.
15. Kaplan DH. In vivo function of Langerhans cells and dermal dendritic cells. Trends Immunol. 2010;31(12):446–51.
16. Vinish M, Cui W, Stafford E, Bae L, Hawkins H, Cox R, et al. Dendritic cells modulate burn wound healing by enhancing early proliferation. Wound Repair Regen. 2016;24(1):6–13.
17. Yanez DA, Lacher RK, Vidyarthi A, Colegio OR. The role of macrophages in skin homeostasis. Pflugers Arch. 2017;469(3–4):455–63.
18. Penn JW, Grobbelaar AO, Rolfe KJ. The role of the TGF-β family in wound healing, burns and scarring: a review. Int J Burns Trauma. 2012;2(1):18–28.
19. Nguyen AV, Soulika AM. The dynamics of the skin's immune system. Int J Mol Sci. 2019;20(8).
20. Long H, Zhang G, Wang L, Lu Q. Eosinophilic skin diseases: a comprehensive review. Clin Rev Allergy Immunol. 2016;50(2):189–213.
21. Charles A, Janeway PT, Mark W, Mark S. Immunology: spektrum; 2002.
22. Escoter-Torres L, Caratti G, Mechtidou A, Tuckermann J, Uhlenhaut NH, Vettorazzi S. Fighting the fire: mechanisms of inflammatory gene regulation by the glucocorticoid receptor. Front Immunol. 2019;10:1859.
23. Michael R. Warner CC. Topical corticosteroids. In: Wolverton comprehensive dermatologic drug therapy, vol. 3. Elsevier; 2013.
24. Cronstein BN, Kimmel SC, Levin RI, Martiniuk F, Weissmann G. A mechanism for the anti-inflammatory effects of corticosteroids: the glucocorticoid receptor regulates leukocyte adhesion to endothelial cells and expression of endothelial-leukocyte adhesion molecule 1 and intercellular adhesion molecule 1. Proc Natl Acad Sci U S A. 1992;89(21):9991–5.
25. Norris DA. Mechanisms of action of topical therapies and the rationale for combination therapy. J Am Acad Dermatol. 2005;53(1 Suppl 1):S17-25.
26. Luger T, Paller AS, Irvine AD, Sidbury R, Eichenfield LF, Werfel T, et al. Topical therapy of atopic dermatitis with a focus on pimecrolimus. J Eur Acad Dermatol Venereol. 2021;35(7):1505–18.
27. Gutfreund K, Bienias W, Szewczyk A, Kaszuba A. Topical calcineurin inhibitors in dermatology. Part I: Properties, method and effectiveness of drug use. Postepy Dermatol Alergol. 2013;30(3):165–9.
28. Kleinman E, Laborada J, Metterle L, Eichenfield LF. What's new in topicals for atopic dermatitis? Am J Clin Dermatol. 2022;23(5):595–603.
29. Paller AS, Fölster-Holst R, Chen SC, Diepgen TL, Elmets C, Margolis DJ, et al. No evidence of increased cancer incidence in children using topical tacrolimus for atopic dermatitis. J Am Acad Dermatol. 2020;83(2):375–81.
30. Asgari MM, Tsai A-L, Avalos L, Sokil M, Quesenberry CP Jr. Association between topical calcineurin inhibitor use and keratinocyte carcinoma risk among adults with atopic dermatitis. JAMA Dermatol. 2020;156(10):1066–73.
31. Allison AC, Eugui EM. Mycophenolate mofetil and its mechanisms of action. Immunopharmacology. 2000;47(2–3):85–118.
32. Maltzman JS, Koretzky GA. Azathioprine: old drug, new actions. J Clin Invest. 2003;111(8):1122–4.

33. Ghaoui N, Hanna E, Abbas O, Kibbi AG, Kurban M. Update on the use of dapsone in dermatology. Int J Dermatol. 2020;59(7):787–95.
34. Schrezenmeier E, Dörner T. Mechanisms of action of hydroxychloroquine and chloroquine: implications for rheumatology. Nat Rev Rheumatol. 2020;16(3):155–66.
35. Forbat E, Ali FR, Al-Niaimi F. Intravenous immunoglobulins in dermatology. Part 1: biological mechanisms and methods of administration. Clin Exp Dermatol. 2018;43(5):513–7.
36. Haussler MR, Haussler CA, Bartik L, Whitfield GK, Hsieh JC, Slater S, et al. Vitamin D receptor: molecular signaling and actions of nutritional ligands in disease prevention. Nutr Rev. 2008;66(10 Suppl 2):S98-112.
37. Prüfer K, Racz A, Lin GC, Barsony J. Dimerization with retinoid X receptors promotes nuclear localization and subnuclear targeting of vitamin D receptors. J Biol Chem. 2000;275(52):41114–23.
38. Zhang Y, Leung DY, Richers BN, Liu Y, Remigio LK, Riches DW, et al. Vitamin D inhibits monocyte/macrophage proinflammatory cytokine production by targeting MAPK phosphatase-1. J Immunol. 2012;188(5):2127–35.
39. Fukuoka M, Ogino Y, Sato H, Ohta T, Komoriya K, Nishioka K, et al. RANTES expression in psoriatic skin, and regulation of RANTES and IL-8 production in cultured epidermal keratinocytes by active vitamin D3 (tacalcitol). Br J Dermatol. 1998;138(1):63–70.
40. Hussain S, Yates C, Campbell MJ. Vitamin D and systems biology. Nutrients. 2022;14(24).
41. Berbis P. Retinoids: mechanisms of action. Ann Dermatol Venereol. 2010;137(Suppl 3):S97-103.
42. Schick MA, Schlegel N. Clinical Implication of phosphodiesterase-4-inhibition. Int J Mol Sci. 2022;23(3).
43. Pincelli C, Schafer PH, French LE, Augustin M, Krueger JG. Mechanisms underlying the clinical effects of apremilast for psoriasis. J Drugs Dermatol. 2018;17(8):835–40.
44. Esser C, Bargen I, Weighardt H, Haarmann-Stemmann T, Krutmann J. Functions of the aryl hydrocarbon receptor in the skin. Semin Immunopathol. 2013;35(6):677–91.
45. Merk HF. The aryl hydrocarbon receptor as the target structure for new drugs in psoriasis and atopic dermatitis. Hautarzt. 2019;70(12):942–7.
46. Haarmann-Stemmann T, Esser C, Krutmann J. The Janus-Faced role of aryl hydrocarbon receptor signaling in the skin: consequences for prevention and treatment of skin disorders. J Invest Dermatol. 2015;135(11):2572–6.
47. van den Bogaard EH, Bergboer JG, Vonk-Bergers M, van Vlijmen-Willems IM, Hato SV, van der Valk PG, et al. Coal tar induces AHR-dependent skin barrier repair in atopic dermatitis. J Clin Invest. 2013;123(2):917–27.
48. Kurschat P, Rubbert A, Poswig A, Scharffetter-Kochanek K, Krieg T, Hunzelmann N. Treatment of psoriatic arthritis with etanercept. J Am Acad Dermatol. 2001;44(6):1052.
49. Silva D, Secamilli EN, Beleli MV, Massuda JY, Franca A, Magalhães RF. Immunobiologicals in dermatology. An Bras Dermatol. 2022;97(3):275–83.
50. Bieber T. Interleukin-13: targeting an underestimated cytokine in atopic dermatitis. Allergy. 2020;75(1):54–62.
51. Wilson NJ, Boniface K, Chan JR, McKenzie BS, Blumenschein WM, Mattson JD, et al. Development, cytokine profile and function of human interleukin 17-producing helper T cells. Nat Immunol. 2007;8(9):950–7.
52. Silfvast-Kaiser A, Paek SY, Menter A. Anti-IL17 therapies for psoriasis. Expert Opin Biol Ther. 2019;19(1):45–54.
53. Sofen H, Smith S, Matheson RT, Leonardi CL, Calderon C, Brodmerkel C, et al. Guselkumab (an IL-23-specific mAb) demonstrates clinical and molecular response in patients with moderate-to-severe psoriasis. J Allergy Clin Immunol. 2014;133(4):1032–40.
54. Nemmer JM, Kuchner M, Datsi A, Oláh P, Julia V, Raap U, et al. Interleukin-31 signaling bridges the gap between immune cells, the nervous system and epithelial tissues. Front Med. 2021;8.
55. Gresnigt MS, van de Veerdonk FL. Biology of IL-36 cytokines and their role in disease. Semin Immunol. 2013;25(6):458–65.

56. Guntern P, Eggel A. Past, present, and future of anti-IgE biologics. Allergy. 2020;75(10):2491–502.
57. Seif F, Khoshmirsafa M, Aazami H, Mohsenzadegan M, Sedighi G, Bahar M. The role of JAK-STAT signaling pathway and its regulators in the fate of T helper cells. Cell Commun Signal. 2017;15(1):23.
58. Morris R, Kershaw NJ, Babon JJ. The molecular details of cytokine signaling via the JAK/STAT pathway. Protein Sci. 2018;27(12):1984–2009.
59. Bieber T. Novel therapies based on the pathophysiology of atopic dermatitis. J Dtsch Dermatol Ges. 2019;17(11):1150–62.
60. Ytterberg SR, Bhatt DL, Mikuls TR, Koch GG, Fleischmann R, Rivas JL, et al. Cardiovascular and cancer risk with Tofacitinib in rheumatoid arthritis. N Engl J Med. 2022;386(4):316–26.
61. Kinter AL, Godbout EJ, McNally JP, Sereti I, Roby GA, O'Shea MA, et al. The common gamma-chain cytokines IL-2, IL-7, IL-15, and IL-21 induce the expression of programmed death-1 and its ligands. J Immunol. 2008;181(10):6738–46.
62. Sirokay J, Mauch C. Melanoma microenvironment-impact of modern therapies. Dermatologie (Heidelb). 2022;73(12):907–14.

Steroid and Non-steroid Immunomodulators

Jonathan Rick, Devea R. De, and Vivian Y. Shi

Abstract Inflammatory skin disorders are a common problem encountered by dermatologists. There is a large and growing armamentarium of immunomodulators aimed to address these conditions. Selecting the appropriate set of medications can greatly improve disease outcome and minimize side effects. However, the diversity of pharmacologic agents also means that options can be intimidating or overlooked. This chapter seeks to update the reader on immunomodulator options currently on the market and outline their strengths and side-effects. The immunomodulators discussed include topical, intralesional and systemic corticosteroids, topical calcineurin inhibitors (tacrolimus and pimecrolimus), oral PDE4 inhibitor (apremilast), topical PDE4 inhibitors (crisaborole and roflumilast), and topical aryl hydrocarbon receptor agonist (tapinarof). Current formulations, common indications, dosing, and appropriate monitoring considerations are reviewed.

Keywords Steroid · Calcineurin · Phosphodiesterase · Inhibitor · Agonist

1 Introduction

Inflammation is a common factor in many dermatologic conditions and relieving inflammation can promote recovery from these diseases. This has spurred the development of numerous medications that are able to attenuate pathological immune responses through a variety of mechanisms. This diversity of approaches allows treatments to be specifically tailored to a patient's needs and provide a favorable

J. Rick
Department of Dermatology, University of California-Davis, Sacramento, CA, USA

D. R. De
Department of Dermatology, Donald and Barbara Zucker School of Medicine at Hofstra/Northwell, New Hyde Park, NY, USA

V. Y. Shi (✉)
Department of Dermatology, University of Washington, Seattle, WA, USA

N. Bhatia (ed.), *Immunomodulators and Biologics in Dermatologic Treatment*,
https://doi.org/10.1007/978-3-031-66590-5_3

adverse event profile. A broad division that is often considered early is the separation of topical or systemic modalities. Some medications can be applied to areas directly affected by disease and therefore reduce the systemic impact of their use. However, patients with extensive disease and extracutaneous symptoms may be poor candidates for this angle of treatment.

2 Corticosteroids

Since the discovery of hydrocortisone in 1952, corticosteroids have undergone tremendous development to alter their potency and specificity [1]. This refinement has created a spectrum of agents that variably activate mineralocorticoid and glucocorticoid receptors [1–3]. The medical application of these substances is broad, but in dermatology the glucocorticoid effects are desired, and these are measured to evaluate steroid potency.

All steroids are derived from cholesterol molecules and consist of three hexane and one pentane ring [1, 4, 5] Modifications to this structure are responsible for altering the potency of these agents to either glucocorticoid or mineralocorticoid receptors. When controlling inflammation, glucocorticoid effects are desired and are responsible for both the rapid and durable reductions in inflammation. Mineralocorticoid effects are responsible for ion shifts between cells and their use can be complex in systemic formulations owning to the need to monitor electrolytes and fluid shifts. Potency is partially determined by lipophilicity as steroids are able to diffuse past plasma membranes to interact with cytoplasmic receptors. These intracellular receptors are responsible for modifying genetic expression patterns responsible for inflammatory disorders and are called the genomic effects. However, membrane-bound receptors are also known to bind glucocorticoids and downregulate cAMP expression to reduce inflammation as well. This more immediate response is still being elucidated, but reductions in cAMP are thought to reduce immediate cell signaling by decreasing the activity of the MEK1/2 pathway and lowering responsiveness to and secretion of stress cytokines [6].

Steroids can be broadly divided into topical or systemic formulations discussed below. A notable deviation from this categorization is the use of intralesional steroids. The most common agent used is triamcinolone, which is routinely available in concentrations as potent as 40 mg/ml [7, 8]. However, this concentration has high risks of dermal atrophy and dilutions down to 2.5 mg/ml are used for more sensitive areas. Thick and/or highly inflamed lesions such as keloids, inflammatory alopecia, prurigo nodularis may benefit most from potent injections (20–40 mg/ml) whereas small lesions in cosmetically important areas are best treated with low concentrations (2.5 mg/ml) [9]. The volumes of injection are often determined by the size of the lesion with large keloids sometimes best treated with several ml, but small inflammatory papules requiring 0.1–0.2 ml.

2.1 Topical Steroids (TCS)

Topical steroids (TCS) have numerous applications for inflammatory cutaneous diseases. Like all topicals, TCS must be able to penetrate cutaneous barriers to affect the tissue underneath. This is achieved by the vehicle that suspends the active ingredient [10, 11]. Vehicles are not inert substances, but instead affect the bioavailability of TCS and may provide chemical substitutions that further drive potency. These mechanisms are complex and are responsible for potency variations that are seen in TCS formulations. TCS can be found suspended in ointments, creams, lotions, gels, foams, tapes/bandages, and solutions, etc. Each of these formulations have specific use cases. Ointments are often preferred when a greasier substance is needed and solutions/gels are preferred when a more water-soluble and absorptive treatment in indicated. However, these suspensions also effect potency. Solutions are thin vehicles that can be applied to regions where a quick-drying and minimally viscus substance is desired.

As TCS are often applied locally, their side-effects are often limited to sites of application [12]. However, applications to large surface areas may promote systemic uptake and induce the systemic side-effects discussed below. Local side-effects can include exacerbation of cutaneous infections by local immunosuppressive effects, folliculitis, dermal atrophy, hypo/hyperpigmentation and hypertrichosis. Rarely, patients may have an allergy to the TCS or vehicles that contain them. Overall, the side-effects to TCS are uncommon if used appropriately and can often be mitigated by limiting their use to locations of active disease, prescribing the appropriate steroid potency, and educating patients on appropriate duration of use. For treating chronic, remitting-relapsing inflammatory dermatoses, patients should be instructed to dynamically escalate and de-escalate the intensity of their treatment based on disease activity. For example, it may be best to start a super-potent agent to quickly control disease flares and then downregulate to mid-potency options. Alternatively, patients may be counselled to take breaks in treating chronic but milder disease as to allow the skin to recover from the side-effects of treatment. Dermal atrophy is of special concern in areas with thinner epidermal barriers and less baseline dermal substance. Steroid atrophy can be experienced in as little as 1–2 weeks of regular super-potent topical steroid use and special precautions should be taken when prescribing them.

TCS are organized base on potency and this scale should be considered when devising treatment plans. Table 1 reviews a selected list of TCS that may be considered and their potency. On body surfaces that naturally have significant dermal substance and thick stratum corneum, more potent medications can be considered [10, 13]. In diseases that have substantial inflammation, produce induration, and or are covered in thick scale, super potent TCS may be ideal to arrest disease. On the other end of the spectrum, mild disease in sensitive areas is best addressed with low potency medications. These areas include the thin flexural surfaces of the axilla, neck and groin, but also cosmetically important areas like the neck and face. Infants and children, which have thin and developing skin, are often best served with less potent formulations as well. Treatments are commonly prescribed daily or twice a day. More frequent treatment is often not more effective and instead likely to create tachyphylaxis and a reduction in disease response [14]. If additional potency is needed, TCS can be applied under an occluding barrier to promote uptake into the skin and reduce loss of topical medication. Fingertip units (FTU) is a favored metric for prescribing steroid volume. The average adult male can hold about 0.5 g of topical steroid on their distal fingertip and this can be used to guide patients as to how much medication should be applied to their body.

2.2 *Systemic Steroids*

Systemic steroids have broad applications in dermatology and are used to treat many inflammatory diseases [15–17]. Although these medications are able to quickly reduce inflammation throughout the body, they are limited by their numerous side-effects. Therefore, systemic steroids are used most commonly for flares of immune-related diseases such as atopic dermatitis, psoriasis, lupus, bullous pemphigoid, and related chronic conditions. Owing to the wide variety of off-target effects, they are often poor choices for the chronic management of immune diseases and steroid-sparing options should be considered early in a patient workup.

Systemic steroids can be given intravenously, intramuscularly or orally. The systemic absorption from intralesional or topical applications is thought to be minimal. When selecting a systemic steroid, consideration is owed to the effect duration (half-life), extent of mineralocorticoid effects, treatment duration and potency. Owing to its potent glucocorticoid effects, mild mineralocorticoid effects, moderate duration of action, and moderate strength; prednisone is the most used systemic steroid in dermatology. The dosing of prednisone depends on the severity of disease being treated. A dose of 0.5 mg/kg is considered a moderate dose and 1.0–3.0 mg/kg is considered a high dose. Most prescriptions will fall into the high dose or moderate dose category.

Steroids are best used for the shortest possible duration. The probability and severity of side-effects rises linearly with dosing. However, for patients requiring long-term steroid use, down titration is needed to prevent adrenal endocrine collapse [16]. All systemic steroids elicit negative feedback on the adrenal axis such that patients no longer produce physiologic amounts of endogenous steroid. The exact duration as to when a taper is required is under debate, but it is generally advised after three weeks of continuous moderate-to-high dose prednisone use. The duration and pattern of titration is not well formalized. A commonly used algorithm is to reduce the total dose of prednisone by 10 mg every 3 days until the patient is at a total dose of 10 mg, at this point 5 mg is used for one week and lastly 2.5 mg for one week. However, other algorithms include decreasing by 10% every 2–3 days until at a physiologic 2.5–5 mg per day. Tapering too rapidly can result in adrenal crisis and/or flaring of the treated condition. However, slow tapers increase steroid exposure and increase the possibility of side-effects. For patients on steroids for over a year,

Table 1 Selected list of common topical steroids sorted by their potency

Potency class	Generic name	Vehicle	Concentration (%)
1	Clobetasol propionate	Lotion, Cream, Solution, Ointment	0.05
	Betamethasone dipropionate	Gel, Ointment	0.05
	Halobetasol propionate	Cream, Ointment	0.05
2	Betamethasone dipropionate	Cream, Ointment	0.05
	Mometasone furoate	Ointment	0.1
	Halcinonide	Ointment, Cream	0.1
	Fluocinonide	Cream, Gel, Ointment	0.05
	Desoximetasone	Cream, Gel, Ointment	0.05/0.025
3	Triamcinolone acetonide	Ointment	0.1
	Fluticasone propionate	Ointment	0.0005
	Betamethasone dipropionate	Cream	0.05
	Fluocinonide	Cream	0.05
	Betamethasone valerate	Foam, Cream, Lotion, Ointment	0.1
4	Triamcinolone acetonide	Cream, Ointment, Spray	0.1
	Mometasone furoate	Cream	0.1
	Fluocinolone acetonide	Ointment	0.025
	Betamethasone benzoate	Gel	0.025
	Hydrocortisone valerate	Ointment	0.2
5	Flurandronolide	Cream, Lotion, Tape	0.05
	Fluticasone propionate	Cream	0.05
	Desonide	Ointment	0.05
	Betamethasone dipropionate	Lotion	0.05
	Triamcinolone acetonide	Lotion	0.1
	Hydrocortisone	Cream	0.1
	Fluocinolone acetonide	Cream	0.025
	Betamethasone benzoate	Cream, Lotion	0.025
	Betamethasone valerate	Cream, Ointment	0.1
	Hydrocortisone valerate	Cream	0.2
6	Fluocinolone acetonide	Oil, Cream, Solution	0.01
	Desonide	Cream	0.05
	Betamethasone valerate	Lotion	0.1
7	Hydrocortisone	Cream	1

Table 2 Non-steroid immunomodulators

Class	Drug name	Topical versus systemic	Formulation	Concentration	Approved conditions	Ongoing trials (latest phase)	Side-effects
Calcineurin inhibitor	Tacrolimus[a]	Topical	Ointment	0.03% or 0.1%	Moderate to severe atopic dermatitis	–	Application site irritation, worsening of herpes simplex virus activation, headache, stomach ache, flu-like symptoms
	Pimecrolimus[b]	Topical	Cream	1%	Mild to moderate atopic dermatitis	–	
PDE4 inhibitor	Apremilast[c]	Systemic	Tablet	10, 20, 30 mg tablets	Psoriasis and Behcet's disease	Atopic dermatitis (phase 2)[d]	Diarrhea, nausea, upper respiratory infection, headache, vomiting, fatigue, decreased appetite, insomnia, backpain, weight loss, depression, tooth ache, folliculitis
	Crisaborole[e]	Topical	Ointment	2%	Psoriasis, mild to moderate atopic dermatitis	–	Application site irritation, cutaneous allergic reaction

(continued)

Table 2 (continued)

Class	Drug name	Topical versus systemic	Formulation	Concentration	Approved conditions	Ongoing trials (latest phase)	Side-effects
	Roflumilast*	Topical	Foam, ointment, cream	0.3%	None	Atopic dermatitis (phase 3)[f], Psoriasis (phase 3)[g]	Pending
Aryl hydrocarbon receptor agonist	Tapinarof*	Topical	Cream	1%	None	Atopic dermatitis (phase 3)[h], Psoriasis (Phase 3)[i]	Pending

[a] *PROTOPIC*®. https://www.accessdata.fda.gov/drugsatfda_docs/label/2011/050777s018lbl.pdf
[b] *Elidel*®. https://www.accessdata.fda.gov/drugsatfda_docs/label/2006/021302s011lbl.pdf
[c] *OTEZLA*®. https://www.accessdata.fda.gov/drugsatfda_docs/label/2019/205437Orig1s007lbl.pdf
[d] Simpson EL, Imafuku S, Poulin Y, et al. A Phase 2 Randomized Trial of Apremilast in Patients with Atopic Dermatitis. *J Invest Dermatol*. 2019;139(5):1063–1072. doi: https://doi.org/10.1016/j.jid.2018.10.043
[e] *EUCRISA*™. https://www.accessdata.fda.gov/drugsatfda_docs/label/2020/207695s007s009s010lbl.pdf
[f] *Trial of PDE4 Inhibition With Roflumilast for the Management of Atopic Dermatitis (INTEGUMENT-II)*. https://clinicaltrials.gov/ct2/show/NCT04773600?term=Roflumilast&cond=Atopic+Dermatitis&draw=2&rank=4. Accessed December 30, 2021
[g] *Trial of PDE4 Inhibition With Roflumilast for the Management of Plaque Psoriasis (DERMIS-1)*. https://clinicaltrials.gov/ct2/show/NCT04211363?term=Roflumilast&cond=Psoriasis&draw=2&rank=7. Accessed December 30, 2021
[h] *Tapinarof for the Treatment of Atopic Dermatitis in Children and Adults*. https://clinicaltrials.gov/ct2/show/NCT05014568?term=Tapinarof&draw=2&rank=6. Accessed December 30, 2021
[i] Lebwohl MG, Stein Gold L, Strober B, et al. Phase 3 Trials of Tapinarof Cream for Plaque Psoriasis. *N Engl J Med*. 2021;385(24):2219–2229. doi: https://doi.org/10.1056/NEJMoa2103629
*Trials and approval still pending, final formulation, concentration and side-effect profiles are not formalized

a two-month taper may be required due to the severe adrenal atrophy that resulted from this medication use.

Moderate and high potency steroid use has a risk of gastric ulcers and gastric ulcer prophylaxis should be considered early in a steroid course [17]. Osteopenia and osteoporosis are other risks for all patients on steroids and calcium/vitamin D supplementation should be considered early as well. Patients with long and high dose steroid courses should be started on antibiotic prophylaxis for infection [18]. A dose of 20 mg/day or greater of prednisone is considered immunosuppressive. Patient specific risk factors should also be evaluated and may be a contraindication to steroids. Poorly controlled diabetes can be precipitated into a hyperglycemic crisis, patient with congestive heart failure can experience rapid fluid shifts. Hypertension can be driven to a hypertensive crisis. Recent myocardial infarction may be complicated by ventricular rupture when steroids are used, psychiatric diseases may be worsened into steroid psychosis and patients with infections may have progression of these diseases. Long-term use of systemic steroids can re-organize adiposity and promote dermal atrophy resulting in a cushingoid habitus of central adiposity and diffuse striae. Therefore, the suitability of a candidate for systemic steroids must be rigorously evaluated.

3 Calcineurin Inhibitors

3.1 Topical Calcineurin Inhibitors (TCIs)

Calcineurin inhibitors are a class of three medications; cyclosporine A, tacrolimus and pimecrolimus; that have similar immunomodulatory mechanisms. The topical calcineurin inhibitors (TCIs), tacrolimus and pimecrolimus, specifically bind to FK506-binding protein which inhibits the proliferation of t-helper cells and reduces inflammatory cytokine expression [19]. The topical formulation of tacrolimus was available in 2000 and pimecrolimus in 2001 [20]. Attempts to make cyclosporine into a topical formulation have not been successful, which is likely due to the larger molecular structure (~650 kDa) exceeding the 500 kDa transdermal diffusion limit. Regardless, pimecrolimus and tacrolimus have enjoyed broad adoption into the dermatology medical arsenal and are used for a number of dermatoses.

Tacrolimus is approved for use in atopic dermatitis (AD), but there are successful reports in use for seborrheic dermatitis, psoriasis, lichen planus, lichen sclerosis, alopecia and vitiligo [21, 22]. Although not formally approved for these other conditions, excellent response has been seen in several of these diseases that rivals topical steroids. They are especially useful in areas with thinner dermis (axilla, neck, perineum) and/or areas that are exceptionally cosmetically sensitive and steroid atrophy is of high concern (e.g. the eyelids, face, perioral region). The lack of steroid side-effects means they are good options for perioral dermatitis and rosacea that flares with steroid applications. For AD specifically, 0.1% tacrolimus appears to be as effective as mid-potency topical steroids [23–26]. Full strength (0.1%) tacrolimus is approved for adults (over 16 years old) who have failed first-line treatment. Current treatment recommendation is twice daily applications to affected areas for three weeks or until lesions are controlled [27]. Once daily application can be done to areas prone to flares to prevent relapse. The 0.03% strength of tacrolimus is approved in children 2–15 years old with similar treatment algorithm recommendations. On the other hand, pimecrolimus is approved for mild to moderate atopic dermatitis and has a potency comparable to 1% hydrocortisone [28]. Although second line, TCIs play an important role in the management of patients with recalcitrant disease. For example, TCIs may be used in conjunction with topical steroids to increase therapeutic effect or offset side-effects of monotherapy with steroids [29].

Topical calcineurin inhibitors have mild side-effect profiles [23]. The most common side-effect is an unpleasant burning sensation that typically fades after repeated applications. The reason for this unpleasant sensation is not well understood and may be due to release of neuropeptides at application from either the medication or vehicle [30]. Several methods may reduce burning at sites of application, including the use of steroids to curb inflammation before applications as TCIs; applying on dry, as opposed moist, skin and maintaining the skin barrier with regular emollient use; and, for adults, taking 500mg of aspirin approximately one hour before TCI application [30]. However, worsening of rosacea, folliculitis, herpes simplex virus, and acne have been reported. Rarely, patients may have a contact allergy. Initial concerns for systemic absorption have not been corroborated by clinical data, but it is generally advised to not apply TCIs to extensive surface areas on patients with severe atopic disease. Both pimecrolimus and tacrolimus are rather large molecules and poorly suited to absorb past cutaneous barriers. The theoretical risks for topical malignancy at site of application, or systemic malignancy due to medical absorption, have not been substantiated. A large study of almost 8000 patients across 9 countries did not identify increased cancer burden in pediatric patients (<16 years old). Nevertheless, the black box warning for this adverse event remains [27, 31].

4 Phosphodiesterase 4 (PDE4) Inhibitors

The first phosphodiesterase 4 (PDE4) inhibitor approved for dermatologic applications was apremilast in 2016 [32]. Since then, other agents have been developed and tested for dermatologic applications. All of these function by inhibiting PDE4, which is an enzyme responsible for breaking down cyclic adenosine monophosphate (cAMP). When PDE4 is inhibited, cAMP levels rise and inflammatory cytokines are subsequently downregulated. Increased cAMP activates PKA, gated ion channels, and proteins of anti-inflammatory cascades that reduce cytokine release. This effect is seen in T-cells, neutrophils and epithelial cells and therefore promote anti-inflammatory effects in many cell types [33, 34].

4.1 Apremilast

Apremilast is currently approved for psoriasis and Bechet's disease in the United States. This oral medication has also been shown to improve other inflammatory disorders such as atopic dermatitis, hidradenitis suppurativa, sarcoidosis and lupus. The first indication for this medication was psoriasis and the most robust improvements are seen in this condition. It is predicted that about 60% of individuals that stay on apremilast will achieve 75% improvement of their psoriasis (PASI75) at 12 weeks [35]. The effects for patients suffering from atopic dermatitis appear to be more middling [36]. A study of apremilast on 191 atopic patients showed no statistical difference in patients treated with 30mg of apremilast twice daily when compared to placebo controls. Attempts to improve clinical response by increasing the dose to 40mg twice a day did result in significant improvement of disease, but were associated with an increased risk of cellulitis.

Many patients (30%) will discontinue apremilast due to side-effects with GI upset being the most common complaint [32]. This may be improved by slowly increasing the dose of apremilast and the medication comes in a starter pack for initiation. However, side-effects of depression, weight loss, fatigue and upper respiratory infections have been reported as well. Of note, apremilast does not have any labeled laboratory monitoring parameters and is not thought to increase risk of tuberculosis infections. It remains a good option for psoriasis patients that would benefit from systemic treatment but are unable to tolerate other systemics or accept injectable medications.

4.2 Crisaborole

Crisaborole was approved for use as a topical treatment for psoriasis in 2016 as a 2% topical ointment [37]. It functions as a general PDE4 inhibitor, but has a preferential inhibition of PDE4B. Clinical trials demonstrated good medical effects that were only limited by mild topical irritation that faded after repeated applications. However, the potency of this agent is limited and most effectively replaces low-to-medium potency topical steroids that are applied to sensitive areas affected by psoriasis, e.g. the axilla, perineum and face. In these areas approximately 70% of patients report improvement, compared to 10% of patients with a vehicle only control, after 1 month of twice daily application [37]. As is the case with apremilast, the effect of crisaborole ointment on atopic dermatitis appears to be less potent than psoriasis [38]. In a phase three clinical trial of mild-to-moderate atopic patients, 33% were cleared or almost cleared with crisaborole after 28 days of twice a day application versus 25% with vehicle controls. Local irritation is the only notable side-effect for atopic patients as well and often faded after a day of continuous application. It is yet to be determined if crisaborole is effective as a topical medication to other conditions.

4.3 *Roflumilast*

Roflumilast is a PDE4 inhibitor that is currently approved for chronic obstructive pulmonary disease as an oral formulation [39]. It is estimated to be 300× more potent than apremilast and it is being studied as a topical agent [40–42]. Preliminary reports have suggested statistically significant improvement in both psoriasis and atopic dermatitis in as early as 4 weeks with daily application, but the full clinical report has not been published (NCT04211363 and NCT04211389). The formulations include a cream, foam, and lotion with intent to study applications for seborrheic dermatitis and vitiligo as well. Although initial reports are promising, real-world efficacy has yet to be established.

5 Aryl Hydrocarbon Receptor (AhR) Agonist

Tapinarof is the prototypic aryl hydrocarbon receptor (AhR) agonist. Tapinarof binds to intracytoplasmic AhR in keratinocytes and cutaneous immune cells where it produces a broad range of effects including activation of the oxidation defense pathway induced by Nuclear Factor E2-related Factor 2(NRF2).Via NRF2 and other related mechanisms, skin barrier genes (namely filaggrin) and anti-inflammatory programs are activated and Th17 expression is downregulated [43]. A phase 3 study in psoriasis and phase 2b study in atopic dermatitis demonstrated disease improvements at 12 weeks when tapinarof 1% cream was applied twice daily [44, 45]. Trials have demonstrated a favorable tolerability profile with the most common side effects being application site irritation and headaches. Although this is a promising new avenue of treatment, the comparative efficacy of tapinarof to other agents, or how it will integrate into treatment algorithms, is yet to be elucidated.

6 Conclusion

Steroids, calcineurin inhibitors, PD4 inhibitors and AhR agonists are valuable tools in the management of inflammatory cutaneous diseases. There is great interest in developing more targeted and more potent medications with favorable side-effect trials which is reflected in this growing body of medications. The diversity of options means that treatments can be tailored to specific patient needs based on their tolerance, extent of disease and comorbid conditions. The management of inflammatory dermatoses is often ongoing and a patient's needs may evolve with time. Familiarity with the full spectrum of medications presented here will equip the practicing dermatologist with a useful toolset.

References

1. Williams DM. Clinical pharmacology of corticosteroids. Respir Care. 2018;63(6):655–70. https://doi.org/10.4187/RESPCARE.06314.
2. Spada F, Barnes TM, Greive KA. Comparative safety and efficacy of topical mometasone furoate with other topical corticosteroids. Australas J Dermatol. 2018;59(3):e168–74. https://doi.org/10.1111/AJD.12762.
3. Oakley R, Arents BWM, Lawton S, Danby S, Surber C. Topical corticosteroid vehicle composition and implications for clinical practice. Clin Exp Dermatol. 2021;46(2):259–69. https://doi.org/10.1111/CED.14473.
4. Stahn C, Buttgereit F. Genomic and nongenomic effects of glucocorticoids. Nat Clin Pract Rheumatol. 2008;4(10):525–33. https://doi.org/10.1038/ncprheum0898.
5. Panettieri RA, Schaafsma D, Amrani Y, Koziol-White C, Ostrom R, Tliba O. Non-genomic effects of glucocorticoids: an updated view. Trends Pharmacol Sci. 2019;40(1):38–49. https://doi.org/10.1016/J.TIPS.2018.11.002.
6. Lösel R, Wehling M. Nongenomic actions of steroid hormones. Nat Rev Mol Cell Biol. 2003;4(1):46–55. https://doi.org/10.1038/nrm1009.
7. Pariser H, Murray PF. Intralesional injections of triamcinolone. Effects of different concentrations on psoriatic lesions. Arch Dermatol. 1963;87(2):183–7. https://doi.org/10.1001/ARCHDERM.1963.01590140045008.
8. Ben Simon GJ, Huang L, Nakra T, Schwarcz RM, McCann JD, Goldberg RA. Intralesional triamcinolone acetonide injection for primary and recurrent chalazia: is it really effective? Ophthalmology. 2005;112(5):913–7. https://doi.org/10.1016/j.ophtha.2004.11.037.
9. Gallagher T, Taliercio M, Nia JK, Hashim PW, Zeichner JA. Dermatologist Use of Intralesional Triamcinolone in the Treatment of Acne. J Clin Aesthet Dermatol. 2020;13(12):41. /pmc/articles/PMC7819588/. Accessed 23 Dec 2021.
10. Kuehl B, Shear NH. The evolution of topical formulations in psoriasis. Skin Therapy Lett. 2018;23(4):5–9. https://pubmed-ncbi-nlm-nih-gov.libproxy.uams.edu/30086183/. Accessed 12 Dec 2021.
11. Ference JD, Last AR. Choosing topical corticosteroids. Am Fam Physician. 2009;79(2):135–40. www.aafp.org/afpAmericanFamilyPhysician135. Accessed 12 Dec 2021.
12. Abraham A, Roga G. Topical steroid-damaged skin. Indian J Dermatol. 2014;59(5):456. https://doi.org/10.4103/0019-5154.139872.
13. Lebwohl M. Psoriasis. Ann Intern Med. 2018;168(7):ITC49–64. https://doi.org/10.7326/AITC201804030.
14. du Vivier A. Tachyphylaxis to topically applied steroids. Arch Dermatol. 1976;112(9):1245–8. https://doi.org/10.1001/ARCHDERM.112.9.1245.
15. Yu SH, Drucker AM, Lebwohl M, Silverberg JI. A systematic review of the safety and efficacy of systemic corticosteroids in atopic dermatitis. J Am Acad Dermatol. 2018;78(4):733-740.e11. https://doi.org/10.1016/J.JAAD.2017.09.074.
16. Zoorob R, Cender D. A different look at corticosteroids. Am Fam Physician. 1998;58(2):443.
17. Liu D, Ahmet A, Ward L, et al. A practical guide to the monitoring and management of the complications of systemic corticosteroid therapy. Allergy Asthma Clin Immunol. 2013;9(1):30. https://doi.org/10.1186/1710-1492-9-30.
18. Coutinho AE, Chapman KE. The anti-inflammatory and immunosuppressive effects of glucocorticoids, recent developments and mechanistic insights. Mol Cell Endocrinol. 2011;335(1):2–13. https://doi.org/10.1016/J.MCE.2010.04.005.
19. Bram RJ, Hung DT, Martin PK, Schreiber SL, Crabtree GR. Identification of the immunophilins capable of mediating inhibition of signal transduction by cyclosporin A and FK506: roles of calcineurin binding and cellular location. Mol Cell Biol. 1993;13(8):4760–9. https://doi.org/10.1128/MCB.13.8.4760-4769.1993.
20. Gutfreund K, Bienias W, Szewczyk A, Kaszuba A. Topical calcineurin inhibitors in dermatology. Part I: properties, method and effectiveness of drug use. Adv Dermatology Allergol Dermatologii I Alergol. 2013;30(3):165. https://doi.org/10.5114/PDIA.2013.35619.

21. Silny W, Sadowska A, Dańczak-Pazdrowska A, Polańska A. Application of tacrolimus in the treatment of skin diseases other than atopic dermatitis. Adv Dermatology Allergol XXVIII. 2011;1:41–5.
22. Campbell J, Carmena R, Pont V, Millan F, Gimeno E. Vitiligo and tacrolimus. J Am Acad Dermatol. 2005;52(3):P171. https://doi.org/10.1016/J.JAAD.2004.10.701.
23. Reitamo S, Rustin M, Harper J, et al. A 4-year follow-up study of atopic dermatitis therapy with 0.1% tacrolimus ointment in children and adult patients. Br J Dermatol. 2008;159(4):942–51. https://doi.org/10.1111/J.1365-2133.2008.08747.X.
24. Remitz A, Harper J, Rustin M, et al. Long-term safety and efficacy of tacrolimus ointment for the treatment of atopic dermatitis in children. Acta Derm Venereol. 2007;87(1):54–61. https://doi.org/10.2340/00015555-0167.
25. Reitamo S, Harper J, Dbos J, et al. 0.03% Tacrolimus ointment applied once or twice daily is more efficacious than 1% hydrocortisone acetate in children with moderate to severe atopic dermatitis: results of a randomized double-blind controlled trial. Br J Dermatol. 2004;150(3):554–62. https://doi.org/10.1046/J.1365-2133.2004.05782.X.
26. Sehgal VN, Srivastava G, Dogra S. Tacrolimus in dermatology-pharmacokinetics, mechanism of action, drug interactions, dosages, and side effects: part I. Skinmed. 2008;7(1):27–30. https://doi.org/10.1111/J.1540-9740.2007.06485.X.
27. Fda. Medication guide protopic® [pro-TOP-ik] (tacrolimus).
28. Paller AS, Lebwohl M, Fleischer AB, et al. Tacrolimus ointment is more effective than pimecrolimus cream with a similar safety profile in the treatment of atopic dermatitis: results from 3 randomized, comparative studies. J Am Acad Dermatol. 2005;52(5):810–22. https://doi.org/10.1016/J.JAAD.2004.12.038.
29. Wahn U, Bos JD, Goodfield M, et al. Efficacy and safety of pimecrolimus cream in the long-term management of atopic dermatitis in children. Pediatrics. 2002;110(1 Pt 1). https://doi.org/10.1542/PEDS.110.1.E2.
30. Madsen S, Price KN, Shi VY, Lio PA. Pearls in mitigating application pain of topical nonsteroidal agents. Dermatology. 2020;236(5):477–80. https://doi.org/10.1159/000508771.
31. Paller AS, Fölster-Holst R, Chen SC, et al. No evidence of increased cancer incidence in children using topical tacrolimus for atopic dermatitis. J Am Acad Dermatol. 2020;83(2):375–81. https://doi.org/10.1016/J.JAAD.2020.03.075.
32. Nassim D, Alajmi A, Jfri A, Pehr K. Apremilast in dermatology: a review of literature. Dermatol Ther. 2020;33(6): e14261. https://doi.org/10.1111/DTH.14261.
33. Schafer PH, Truzzi F, Parton A, et al. Phosphodiesterase 4 in inflammatory diseases: effects of apremilast in psoriatic blood and in dermal myofibroblasts through the PDE4/CD271 complex. Cell Signal. 2016;28(7):753–63. https://doi.org/10.1016/J.CELLSIG.2016.01.007.
34. Li H, Zuo J, Tang W. Phosphodiesterase-4 Inhibitors for the treatment of inflammatory diseases. Front Pharmacol. 2018;9(OCT):1048. https://doi.org/10.3389/FPHAR.2018.01048.
35. Papadavid E, Rompoti N, Theodoropoulos K, Kokkalis G, Rigopoulos D. Real-world data on the efficacy and safety of apremilast in patients with moderate-to-severe plaque psoriasis. J Eur Acad Dermatol Venereol. 2018;32(7):1173–9. https://doi.org/10.1111/JDV.14832.
36. Simpson EL, Imafuku S, Poulin Y, et al. A phase 2 randomized trial of apremilast in patients with atopic dermatitis. J Invest Dermatol. 2019;139(5):1063–72. https://doi.org/10.1016/J.JID.2018.10.043.
37. Hashim PW, Chima M, Kim HJ, et al. Crisaborole 2% ointment for the treatment of intertriginous, anogenital, and facial psoriasis: a double-blind, randomized, vehicle-controlled trial. J Am Acad Dermatol. 2020;82(2):360–5. https://doi.org/10.1016/J.JAAD.2019.06.1288.
38. Yosipovitch G, Simpson EL, Tan H, et al. Effect of crisaborole topical ointment, 2%, on atopic dermatitis–associated pruritus: an extended analysis of 2 phase 3 clinical trials. Itch. 2018;3(2):e12–e12. https://doi.org/10.1097/ITX.0000000000000012.
39. Wedzicha JA, Calverley PM, Rabe KF. Roflumilast: a review of its use in the treatment of COPD. Int J Chron Obstruct Pulmon Dis. 2016;11:81–90. https://doi.org/10.2147/COPD.S89849.
40. Lé AM, Torres T. New topical therapies for psoriasis. Am J Clin Dermatol. 2021. https://doi.org/10.1007/S40257-021-00649-W.

41. Trial of PDE4 inhibition with roflumilast for the management of plaque psoriasis—full text view—clinicaltrials.gov. https://clinicaltrials.gov/ct2/show/NCT04211363. Accessed 19 Dec 2021.
42. Lebwohl M, Kircik LH, Moore AY, et al. Once-daily roflumilast cream 0.3%, a potent phosphodiesterase-4 inhibitor, provided safe and effective treatment of psoriasis in the DERMIS-1 and DERMIS-2 Phase 3 Trials. Ski J Cutan Med. 2021;5(6):s42–s42. https://doi.org/10.25251/SKIN.5.SUPP.42.
43. Smith SH, Jayawickreme C, Rickard DJ, et al. Tapinarof is a natural AhR agonist that resolves skin inflammation in mice and humans. J Invest Dermatol. 2017;137(10):2110–9. https://doi.org/10.1016/J.JID.2017.05.004.
44. Paller AS, Stein Gold L, Soung J, Tallman AM, Rubenstein DS, Gooderham M. Efficacy and patient-reported outcomes from a phase 2b, randomized clinical trial of tapinarof cream for the treatment of adolescents and adults with atopic dermatitis. J Am Acad Dermatol. 2021;84(3):632–8. https://doi.org/10.1016/J.JAAD.2020.05.135.
45. Lebwohl MG, Gold LS, Strober B, et al. Phase 3 trials of tapinarof cream for plaque psoriasis. 2021;385(24):2219–29. https://doi.org/10.1056/NEJMOA2103629.

Biologics as Immunomodulators

Jonathan Koptyev and George Han

Abstract The advancements made in the applications of biological therapies in dermatology have been game changing, from diseases needing impactful and directed therapy such as psoriasis and atopic dermatitis to diseases that lacked a successful option such as Hidradenitis Suppurativa and Urticaria. Understanding the mechanisms of action of these therapies helps to define not only their potential but their safety as compared to other systemic immunosuppressants that function in less specific manners. This review of biologics as immunomodulators will underline the specificity of action as the asset for both efficacy and safety.

Keywords Inflammation · Biologic · Psoriasis · Immunogenicity · Inhibitor

1 What Are Biologics and What Are They Made of?

Biologics, or biological products, are biotechnology-derived therapeutics that include product types such as vaccines, blood and blood components, allergenics, somatic cells, gene therapy, tissues, and recombinant therapeutic proteins. These biopharmaceuticals are derived from natural living materials including plants, animals, or microorganisms with the goal of treating, preventing, or curing human disease [1].

The chemical composition of biologics is primarily comprised of proteins containing L-amino acids and carbohydrates. Some biologics contain both a protein moiety and a small molecule component, such as antibody–drug conjugates [2]. As intramolecular interactions can form secondary, tertiary, and even quaternary structures, biologics form complex three-dimensional structures that are sensitive to factors such as pH and temperature [3]. With regard to their size, measured in molecular weight (MW), biologic drugs are much larger than typical small molecule chemical compounds used widely in medicine. Whereas small molecule drugs typically weigh less than 1 kDa, biologic drugs range from a few kDa to 1000 kDa [4]. In addition, biologics have a more complex and heterogeneous molecular structure than

J. Koptyev · G. Han (✉)
Zucker School of Medicine at Hofstra/Northwell, New Hyde Park, NY, USA
e-mail: georgehanmdphd@gmail.com

N. Bhatia (ed.), *Immunomodulators and Biologics in Dermatologic Treatment*,
https://doi.org/10.1007/978-3-031-66590-5_4

do chemical compounds. In contrast to the well-defined structure of chemical drugs, the structural features of biologics *in vivo* are not necessarily well-characterized [2].

2 Biologic Development

The development of biologics, also known as biomanufacturing, is a complex multi-step process. An essential step in biologic development is recombinant DNA technology, which lies at the heart of production of biological drugs. Simply put, this is a biochemical process that isolates DNA from human cells, uniquely modifies it, and inserts it into another organism in order to express it in that organism's genetic material. Further, biologic production requires distinct assays, equipment, and facilities from those involved in the manufacture of small molecule drugs. Changes in any step of the manufacturing process could induce alterations in the final product, namely in its identity, safety, purity, and potency [5].

As these drugs can be extremely sensitive to physical conditions, their production is more expensive and time-consuming, necessitating sophisticated technology and controlled processes. Safety challenges can also present during manufacture, as improper sourcing of biological material can lead to an increased risk of product contamination. Lastly, the regulatory considerations of biologic manufacture are extensive, consisting of high levels of review and oversight. For these reasons, there is a substantial gap in manufacturing capacity and, subsequently, cost differential between biologic and chemical drugs [6]. Nevertheless, many large pharmaceutical companies have pivoted towards biologic drug development as the field has become one of the fastest growing classes of therapeutic compounds.

3 Historical Clinical Use of Biologics

Of particular importance to the clinical arena, biologics are bioengineered to target specific genes or proteins involved in the pathogenesis of disease. Some examples of modern biologics are recombinant therapeutic proteins, such as monoclonal antibodies (mAbs), cytokines, growth factors, enzymes, and immunomodulators. Interestingly, the first human insulin, or "Humulin," was a recombinant therapeutic protein developed in 1982 [7] It is now considered to have been the first biological product approved for general medical use. By the year 2003, there were 140 recombinant proteins developed globally, with an estimated $30 billion market for biological products, and the growth in the biologics market far outpaces that of small molecule drugs [8].

Since then, biologics have been utilized to treat a wide spectrum of organ systems and disease states. Based on results from randomized controlled trials, various medical disciplines have employed biologics in the treatment of chronic and serious diseases, including breast cancer, rheumatoid arthritis, ulcerative colitis, asthma, and anemia. We have seen the discovery of T-cell activation inhibitors/co-stimulation modulators, tumor necrosis factor (TNF) inhibitors, and anti-interleukin drugs, among others [9].

The goal of many biologics is to improve disease-related symptoms and quality of life after traditional chemical drugs have been tried and proven to be ineffective. A biologic could have the attractive feature of being a more targeted treatment modality, avoiding complex discussions of risk vs. benefit that can be seen in more broad-acting, narrow therapeutic window small molecule drugs. Disease characteristics such as etiology, lab findings, severity, and risk level are other important factors in the choosing to start biologic therapy. For example, in patients with moderate to severe Crohn's disease, biologic treatment is considered first-line [10]. Other biologics have defined criteria that patients must meet to be eligible for treatment. For instance, only asthma patients with an IgE level $\geq$30 IU/mL with clinical and testing evidence for atopy are considered candidates for omalizumab [11].

4 Pharmacokinetics of Biologics

Since biologic molecules are generally too large to be administered orally without being destroyed before entering the blood stream, they are usually injected or infused. In other words, the oral bioavailability of biologics is extremely low. Bioavailability is defined as the proportion of the drug that is available to exert a therapeutic effect after being introduced to the body. Intravenous administration is the most reliable route of administration with regard to bioavailability, but comes with its own set of challenges (such as the possibility of an infusion reaction) and is the most burdensome to patients. In addition to their size, the inherent instability of the molecular structure of biologics makes it incompatible with a pill form. Although there have been significant advances in oral delivery, no oral biologic is yet available for commercial use [12]. Pulmonary delivery of biologics is another route of administration, as the lungs have a large surface area and high perfusion rate [4]. Other forms of drug delivery that have been utilized are subcutaneous, transdermal, nasal, and buccal routes [13].

As far as distribution of the drug, biologic distribution is usually limited to plasma and/or extracellular fluids. Small molecule drugs, however, can distribute to any combination of organs or tissues and readily cross blood capillary membranes. Since biologics contain larger proteins, they cross blood capillaries more slowly. Distribution can also be affected by specific protein binding, namely to proteins involved in the transport and regulation of the biologic drug [3]. Absorption of biologics depends on molecular weight but is also dependent on other extrinsic factors like depth of injection, blood flow at injection site, exercise, rubbing and temperature [4]. Of course, these complex pharmacokinetic properties must be considered and analyzed during pre-clinical testing.

5 Immunogenicity

One of the most important effects of biologics is their immunogenicity, namely, their ability to provoke an immune response. The formation of anti-drug antibodies (ADAbs) is one of the main mechanisms by which this is seen [14]. As biologics structurally differ from endogenous immunoglobulins, they can lead to the production of ADAbs, which are antibodies produced by the host that are directed against the biologic agent. The extent to which these are produced can depend on the particular structure of the biologic agent and its target molecule, as well as on other factors such as dosing regimen. Importantly, the presence of ADAbs has been found to contribute to biologic treatment failure and increased risk of therapy-limiting adverse events [9].

There are other unintended immunologic consequences of biologics that must be considered when initiating therapy. After all, many of these drugs block physiologic immune pathways that are normally in place to protect the host. Immunosuppression, both within the context of innate and adaptive immunity, is a significant risk of some biologics. Increased risk of bacterial, viral and fungal opportunistic infections, reactivation of latent tuberculosis, reactivation of hepatitis B, and neutropenia are some of the adverse immune-related events seen with biologic administration. Some drugs carry black box warnings related to immunologic side effects, which are important to note for prescribers and patients alike [15].

6 Common Biologic Types

Therapeutic biologics are often made up of immunoglobulin, also known as antibody, products. Generally, antibodies can be classified into five isotypes: IgM, IgD, IgG, IgE and IgA. For therapeutic antibodies, IgG is the predominant isotype, containing two heavy chains and two light chains interconnected via disulfide bonds (Fig. 1). Each chain has an N-terminal variable region and a C-terminal constant region. On each variable region of each pair of heavy and light chains are hypervariable loops called complementarity determining regions (CDRs). This forms the antigen binding region at the end of the IgG protein [16].

While most antibodies produced by the normal immune response are polyclonal, meaning that they come from a number of different B lymphocytes, it is possible to produce large numbers of a single antibody from one B-cell line, rendering the antibody monoclonal [17]. Monoclonal antibodies (mAbs), representing the largest class of biologic drugs, have been a widely used type of biologic in the treatment of immunologic diseases and cancer [2]. They are designed to have a specific antigen recognition site and robust affinity to target proteins and subsequently achieve the desired downstream effect. Because their affinities are so exquisite, with ability to bind to targets in the picomolar to nanomolar range, this often translates into low off-target toxicity [18]. mAbs are homogenous products in that every antibody in the

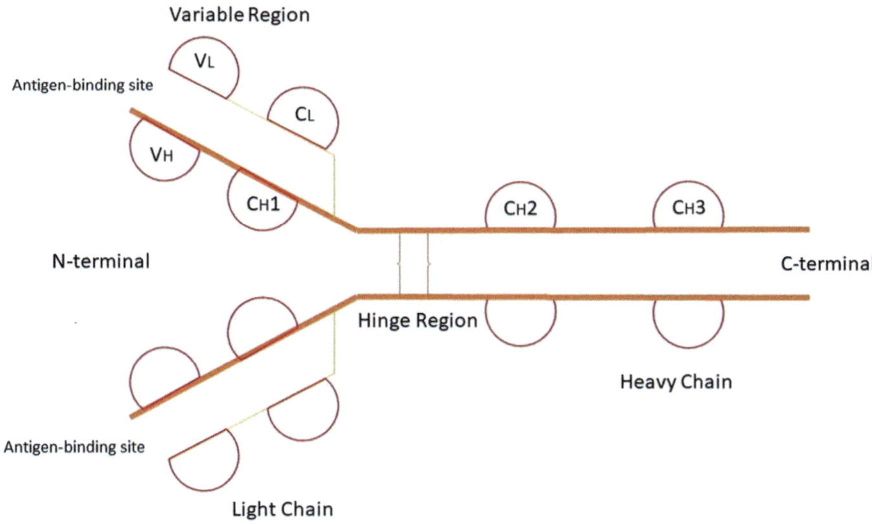

Fig. 1 Basic structure of IgG molecule

preparation is identical in sequence and has the same antigen recognition site. Polyclonal antibodies, however, have different protein sequences and recognize various epitopes on an antigen [17].

mAbs derived from nonhuman sources can be "humanized" through recombinant DNA technologies, which essentially makes their amino acid sequence more similar to that of humans. Humanized mAbs usually contain small parts of their CDR that are obtained from nonhuman sources, and larger constant regions of the immunoglobulin heavy and light chains that are human-derived. This is typically done to reduce the mAb's immunogenicity, as the more similar a mAb is to shared human sequences, the less likely it is to induce the host immune response against it. Chimeric antibodies are another type of humanized antibody that contain a larger portion of nonhuman protein sequence [16]. Zenapax (daclizumab) was the first FDA-approved humanized antibody in 1997 used to prevent renal allograft rejection [2].

Antibody fragments, instead of whole antibodies, can also be used to enhance the drug's pharmacokinetics and distribution into tissue [19]. Fragments have a single antigen binding site rather than the two that are typically seen with whole antibodies. Fragment antigen-binding (Fab) fragments, are one example of this concept. They lack the Fc component of the original antibody, consisting only of a variable domain and the first constant region of each heavy and light chain. These are generated by papain digestion of whole IgG antibodies, which removes the entire Fc portion as well as the hinge region. Abciximab is a F_{ab} fragment therapeutic that binds to the platelet glycoprotein IIb/IIIa receptor and inhibits platelet aggregation.

Another mAb variant is the F_c fusion protein. The F_c portion of an antibody can be fused to another protein fragment such as the extracellular domain of a cell surface receptor. Although fusion proteins do not have a CDR, they manipulate the specific function of the protein to which they are fused. Etanercept is a fusion-based biologic that consists of the combination of two TNF-α receptors with the F_c portion of IgG. Binding to TNF-α bivalently, Etanercept is used to inhibit the role of TNF-α in disease states [20].

7 Common Biologic Mechanisms

As noted above, biologics can function through various mechanisms. It is important to distinguish between their distinct targets, as some biologics bind to cell surface antigens whereas others bind to cytoplasmic targets. In some cases, the drug can target a cell surface receptor, blocking its normal ligand from binding the receptor. This interruption of physiologic receptor function may in turn prevent cell proliferation or survival, for instance. Other potential drug targets include cancer cells, B-lymphocytes, plasma proteins, growth factors, bacteria and viruses [21].

Importantly for inflammatory disease processes, biologic agents are typically engineered to bind and inhibit inflammatory cytokines that are implicated in pathogenesis, which has numerous benefits. First cytokines that have been identified to mediate the inflammatory process can be precisely studied and targeted. The role of cytokines in disease can be investigated using animal models, which provides an advantage in research and drug discovery. At the same time, targeting cytokines can be challenging for several reasons. Cytokines function by a compensatory system called redundancy, in which the effects achieved by blocking one cytokine's activity can be compensated by others. In addition, cytokines are known to be pleiotropic, meaning that they influence several processes simultaneously, including a normal immune response [22]. As such, finding an appropriate target to block with a cytokine that inhibits enough of an immunologic process to control a disease state is challenging, but important.

8 Applications of Biologics in Dermatology

For the field of dermatology, biologics have been a beneficial addition to the treatment repertoire for inflammatory skin disease. The first biologic used for a dermatologic condition was alefacept, which was introduced in the year 2003 for treatment of psoriasis and psoriatic arthritis [23]. Being a biologic targeting activation of T cells, the risk–benefit profile was not attractive compared to newer agents which soon came to market, and the drug was withdrawn several years later. As biologic drug production has greatly developed over the years, the field of psoriasis therapeutics has since seen the addition of many more biologic drug treatment options, including adalimumab, etanercept, infliximab, certolizumab, ixekizumab, secukinumab, brodalumab, ustekinumab, guselkumab, tildrakizumab, and risankizumab as of 2022 [24]. Moreover, biologics have been utilized for the management of many other dermatologic diseases, in some cases off-label. Many of these diseases have become more manageable with biologics as these drugs have provided a new hope for many patients with severe and recalcitrant symptoms.

9 Psoriasis

Psoriasis is an immune-mediated disease that can involve the skin and joints, affecting 0.51–3.2% of the United States population [25]. While there are specific criteria to consider, generally patients with moderate to severe plaque psoriasis who are candidates for systemic immunomodulator therapy (including older oral medications such as methotrexate and cyclosporine) can be assessed for biologic treatment [24]. Clinical data for psoriasis has shown that biologic agents are effective in improving symptoms and have a relatively good safety profile for long-term use [23]. As several immune mediators have been implicated in playing a role in the pathogenesis of psoriasis, there are numerous important targets for treatment and thus classes of medications targeting psoriasis [26].

There is a considerable history behind our understanding of the pathogenesis of psoriasis, however, that must first be elucidated in order to better grasp the modern-day application of biologics. To begin, in 2005, there was a thought that psoriasis pathophysiology was mediated by a type 1 pathway driven by T lymphocytes, Th1 and Tc1 cells in particular [27] Later, a 2008 clinical trial showed that, in addition to Th1 cells, T helper type 17 (Th17) cells played a role in disease, specifically in epidermal activation [28]. As psoriasis research progressed, interleukin (IL) 22 and 23 were also implicated [29]. Overall, the present view on psoriasis immune pathogenesis is centered around an IL-23 and IL-17 pathway, where an activated dendritic cell leads to increased IL-23 production, which in turn stimulates Th17 cells to produce more IL-17, leading to keratinocyte hyperproliferation and an inflammatory feedback loop [30].

Parallel to the evolution of our understanding of psoriasis pathogenesis over the past two decades, our treatment paradigms have changed as well. Early targeting of TNF-α marked its role as a major cytokine driving inflammation in psoriasis. As part of the innate immune system, TNF-α has a variety of functions such as increasing production of pro-inflammatory and adhesion molecules [31]. It has been found to often be elevated in patients with psoriasis [32]. Importantly, the significance of TNF-α in psoriasis has been demonstrated through the many clinical trials that have used anti-TNF-α biologic drugs for psoriasis treatment. Each anti-TNF-α drug has a different mechanism by which it inhibits the cytokine. As mentioned previously, etanercept is an example of a fusion-based biologic that competitively binds and mimics the TNF-α receptor [33]. Infliximab, on the other hand, binds to soluble and transmembrane forms of TNF-α with high affinity and is given intravenously, rather than subcutaneously as with the other psoriasis biologics [34].

IL-17 is another cytokine that is targeted by many psoriasis biologics. In keratinocytes, or skin cells, IL-17 stimulates the production of antimicrobial peptides, proinflammatory cytokines and chemokines, and pro-proliferative cytokines [35]. An anti-IL17 drug such as secukinumab binds and neutralizes IL-17A, a cytokine of the IL-17 family [36]. Similarly, other drugs selectively bind IL-23, a proinflammatory cytokine responsible for the differentiation and proliferation of Th17 cells. By binding to IL-23's p19 subunit, biologic drugs such as guselkumab and tildrakizumab can inhibit the Th17-related cascade promoted by IL-23 [26].

10 Other Applications of Biologics in Dermatology

Current research and application of biologic drugs within dermatology have extended far beyond their origins in psoriasis. Our traditional biologic drugs for psoriasis have found uses in diseases such as hidradenitis suppurativa (HS), granuloma annulare (GA), pyoderma gangrenosum (PG), cutaneous sarcoidosis (CS), and others. As we will soon establish, through similar therapeutic mechanisms, these same drugs can be applicable to inflammatory dermal conditions, autoimmune bullous skin disease as well as disorders of follicular occlusion.

HS is a chronic inflammatory skin condition of the apocrine glands, causing persistent or recurrent nodules and abscesses that lead to the formation of sinus tracts and scarring. There is widespread evidence of treatment effectiveness of both infliximab and adalimumab, two anti-TNF-α biologics [37]. Fortunately, adalimumab has been the first FDA-approved drug for treatment of HS. Newer reports and studies of HS treatment with ustekinumab, an IL-12/23 pathway inhibitor [38], have also shown promising results. Blok and colleagues conducted a small uncontrolled open-label clinical trial in 2015 of 17 HS patients treated with ustekinumab in which 12 subjects completed the protocol, of which 82% had moderate to marked improvement of skin lesions in the primary outcome by week 40 of treatment [39].

Granuloma annulare is another condition in which biologic treatment has shown benefit. GA is described clinically as smooth annular papules and plaques that show necrobiotic granulomas on histology. A 2016 single-center observational study published in the Journal of the American Academy of Dermatology (JAAD) suggested that adalimumab could be effective for patients with GA, especially those who have generalized or disseminated disease [40]. Other reports showed clearing of GA with infliximab, while etanercept had mixed results [41–44]. This use of TNF-α inhibitors for GA is in line with a study that found that overexpression of TNF-α by peripheral mononuclear lymphocytes and macrophages may play a role in GA development [45]. In addition, it is well known that granulomas are mostly made up of mononuclear cells with lymphocytes and macrophages secreting TNF-α and interferon-gamma.

Pyoderma gangrenosum is an autoinflammatory disease belonging to the group of neutrophilic dermatoses that presents as an enlarging, non-healing full-thickness ulcer. Infliximab, ustekinumab, and canakinumab (an IL-1β inhibitor) have all been used for the treatment of PG [46–49]. Other TNF-α inhibitors—etanercept and adalimumab—have also been used, with mixed results. A more balanced treatment approach may be necessary when considering biologics for PG, depending on the extent of disease size and severity.

Cutaneous sarcoidosis, the skin manifestations of a multisystem granulomatous disease, has also been treated with TNF-α inhibitors. Many case reports and studies have reported positive results with biologics such as infliximab and adalimumab [50–55]. Since CS is also granulomatous, similar to GA is, there is pathogenic involvement of TNF-α, namely in its role in granuloma formation. Nevertheless, it is critical to note the numerous reports of TNF-α antagonists paradoxically causing sarcoid-like disease [56–58].

Other dermatologic conditions that have employed biologic treatment include necrobiosis lipoidica, bullous pemphigoid, pemphigus, alopecia areata, and many others. In this regard, biologic use in dermatology has seen a remarkable increase in application and administration, marking the next phase of this therapeutic era for dermatologists.

11 IL-1 and Autoinflammation

As we have discussed various biologic uses in dermatology, one disease-pathway combination particularly stands out—IL-1β and PG. In this regard, IL-1β has been shown to be a proinflammatory cytokine integral to an autoinflammatory pathway seen in PG. Autoinflammation is defined as heightened neutrophil-predominant inflammation predominantly mediated by cytokines of innate immunity, particularly IL-1β, without the presence of autoantibodies. This differs from autoimmunity, which is a more pronounced defect of adaptive immunity [59]. Autoinflammatory diseases are typically chronic, debilitating syndromes, with many having strong genetic components [60]. In fact, patients with autoinflammatory syndromes have been shown to release more IL-1β from blood monocytes than healthy individuals [61].

Mechanistically, IL-1β requires cleavage of its proform by caspase-1 in order to become active. Discovered in 2002, the inflammasome is a caspase-activating complex comprised of caspase-1, caspase-5, Pycard/Asc, and NALP1 [62]. The inflammosome regulates immunologic responses to both exogenous and endogenous stimuli that lead to activation of caspase-1, i.e. pathogens, neoplasia [63]. As such, autoinflammatory pathways are centered around the inflammasome and its role in innate immunity.

With regard to therapies, a common feature of autoinflammatory diseases is response to IL-1 blockade, the effect of drugs such as anakinra, rilonacept and canakinumab [59]. In the skin, the IL-1 family of cytokines has been previously linked to dermatologic conditions such as cutaneous lupus erythematosus, psoriasis (particularly pustular psoriasis), atopic dermatitis and autoimmune bullous diseases [64]. In addition, there is a group of monogenic autoinflammatory diseases such as cryopyrinopathies that present with inflammatory flares of fever and skin lesions. IL-1 antagonists have been a major breakthrough for these disorders as well as for other refractory inflammatory conditions where neutrophils play an important role in the pathogenesis [65].

12 Other Biologics

Other biologics exist in dermatology, such as inhibitors of IL-4 and/or IL-13, dupilumab and tralokinumab. These medications have fundamentally altered our approach to another condition, atopic dermatitis, and have found shared uses in some cases for treating other allergic diseases and asthma as well. Omalizumab has been approved for treating chronic spontaneous urticaria and rituximab is also approved for treatment of pemphigus vulgaris. With each of these conditions, a close linkage between disease state pathogenesis and an appropriate target for which a biologic exists was found. Further research into other skin conditions is ongoing and biosimilars are also another important class of medication to consider. In biosimilars, biologic development has found its equivalent to generic medications, where reverse engineering of a biologic medication is employed to generate a "similar" biologic that can be used in the same disease states the original drug was approved to treat. This is a rapidly developing field of study, and the innovations will no doubt come quickly, so it is prudent to keep abreast of the latest developments in biologic research and manufacture.

13 Conclusion

The advent of biologic therapeutics has greatly contributed to both our understanding and treatment of chronic disease. As immunomodulators, biologics have a wide variety of uses in dermatology, especially in inflammatory skin diseases. More biologic drugs are developed each year, providing new optimism for patients with difficult-to-treat conditions. With such effective treatments available in the form of biologic medications, an understanding of their generation and physiology with the appropriate risks and benefits in mind is important in utilizing these drugs appropriately. This way, providers can strive to ensure that their patients enjoy the benefits of biologics while minimizing the potential harms. We're just at the tip of the iceberg when it comes to biologic medications, and new discoveries are likely to come as scientific breakthroughs continue to arrive in dermatology.

References

1. Center for drug evaluation and research. What are "biologics" questions and answers. U.S. Food & Drug Administration. https://www.fda.gov/about-fda/center-biologics-evaluation-and-research-cber/what-are-biologics-questions-and-answers. Accessed 3 Mar 2022.
2. Wang, Singh M. Biological drug products: development and strategies. Wiley; 2013.
3. Baumann A. Early development of therapeutic biologics–pharmacokinetics. Curr Drug Metab. 2006;7(1):15–21. https://doi.org/10.2174/138920006774832604.
4. Zhao L, Shang EY, Sahajwalla CG. Application of pharmacokinetics-pharmacodynamics/ clinical response modeling and simulation for biologics drug development. J Pharm Sci. 2012;101(12):4367–82. https://doi.org/10.1002/jps.23330.
5. Center for Drug Evaluation and Research. Developing and manufacturing drugs including biologics. U.S. Food and Drug Administration. https://www.fda.gov/drugs/coronavirus-covid-19-drugs/developing-and-manufacturing-drugs-including-biologics. Accessed 3 Mar 2022.
6. Morrow T, Felcone LH. Defining the difference: What makes biologics unique. Biotechnol Healthc. 2004;1(4):24–9.
7. Altman LK. A new insulin given approval for use in U.S. The New York Times. https://www.nytimes.com/1982/10/30/us/a-new-insulin-given-approval-for-use-in-us.html. Published October 30, 1982. Accessed 3 Mar 2022.
8. Walsh G. Second-generation biopharmaceuticals. Eur J Pharm Biopharm. 2004;58(2):185–96. https://doi.org/10.1016/j.ejpb.2004.03.012.
9. Strand V, Balsa A, Al-Saleh J, et al. Immunogenicity of biologics in chronic inflammatory diseases: a systematic review. BioDrugs. 2017;31(4):299–316. https://doi.org/10.1007/s40259-017-0231-8.
10. Sandborn WJ. Crohn's disease evaluation and treatment: clinical decision tool. Gastroenterology. 2014;147(3):702–5. https://doi.org/10.1053/j.gastro.2014.07.022.
11. National Asthma Education and Prevention Program: Expert panel report III: Guidelines for the diagnosis and management of asthma. Bethesda, MD: National Heart, Lung, and Blood Institute; 2007. (NIH publication no. 08-4051) www.nhlbi.nih.gov/guidelines/asthma/asthgdln.htm. Accessed 31 Aug 2021.
12. New R. Oral delivery of biologics via the intestine. Pharmaceutics. 2020;13(1):18. Published 2020 Dec 24. https://doi.org/10.3390/pharmaceutics13010018.
13. Anselmo AC, Gokarn Y, Mitragotri S. Non-invasive delivery strategies for biologics. Nat Rev Drug Discov. 2019;18(1):19–40. https://doi.org/10.1038/nrd.2018.183.
14. Center for Biologics Evaluation and Research. Immunogenicity of protein-based therapeutics. U.S. Food and Drug Administration. https://www.fda.gov/vaccines-blood-biologics/biologics-research-projects/immunogenicity-protein-based-therapeutics. Published June 23, 2020. Accessed 3 Mar 2022.
15. Henrickson SE, Ruffner MA, Kwan M. Unintended immunological consequences of biologic therapy. Curr Allergy Asthma Rep. 2016;16(6):46. https://doi.org/10.1007/s11882-016-0624-7.
16. Male D., Stokes Peebles R., Male V. Immunology, 9th ed. Elsevier; 2021.
17. Lipman NS, Jackson LR, Trudel LJ, Weis-Garcia F. Monoclonal versus polyclonal antibodies: distinguishing characteristics, applications, and information resources. ILAR J. 2005;46(3):258–68. https://doi.org/10.1093/ilar.46.3.258.
18. Kaymakcalan Z, et al. Comparisons of affinities, avidities, and complement activation of adalimumab, infliximab, and etanercept in binding to soluble and membrane tumor necrosis factor. Clin Immunol. 2009;131(2):308–16.
19. Zhao A, Tohidkia MR, Siegel DL, Coukos G, Omidi Y. Phage antibody display libraries: a powerful antibody discovery platform for immunotherapy. Crit Rev Biotechnol. 2016;36(2):276–89. https://doi.org/10.3109/07388551.2014.958978.
20. Pan A, Gerriets V. Etanercept. In: StatPearls. StatPearls Publishing; 2021.

21. Mali A, Sawant A, Mahadik A, Nair S. Immunotherapy for autoimmune diseases. In: Sawarkar SP, Nikam VS, Syed S, editors. Immunotherapy—a novel facet of modern therapeutics. Springer; 2021.
22. Rider P, Carmi Y, Cohen I. Biologics for targeting inflammatory cytokines, clinical uses, and limitations. Int J Cell Biol. 2016;2016:9259646. https://doi.org/10.1155/2016/9259646.
23. Arndt KA, Hsu JTS, Alam M, Bhatia AC, Chilukuri S. Manual of dermatologic therapeutics, 8th ed. Wolters Kluwer; 2014.
24. Smith CH, Jabbar-Lopez ZK, Yiu ZZ, et al. British association of dermatologists guidelines for biologic therapy for psoriasis 2017. Br J Dermatol. 2017;177(3):628–36. https://doi.org/10.1111/bjd.15665.
25. Michalek IM, Loring B, John SM. A systematic review of worldwide epidemiology of psoriasis. J Eur Acad Dermatol Venereology JEADV. 2017;31(2):205–12. https://doi.org/10.1111/jdv.13854.
26. de Alcantara CC, Reiche EMV, Simão ANC. Cytokines in psoriasis. Adv Clin Chem. 2021;100:171–204. https://doi.org/10.1016/bs.acc.2020.04.004.
27. Krueger JG, Bowcock A. Psoriasis pathophysiology: current concepts of pathogenesis. Ann Rheum Dis. 2005;64(Suppl 2):ii30–6. https://doi.org/10.1136/ard.2004.031120.
28. Zaba LC, Cardinale I, Gilleaudeau P, et al. Amelioration of epidermal hyperplasia by TNF inhibition is associated with reduced Th17 responses [published correction appears in J Exp Med. 2008;205(8):1941. Suárez Fariñas, Mayte [corrected to Suárez-Fariñas, Mayte]]. J Exp Med. 2007;204(13):3183–94. https://doi.org/10.1084/jem.20071094.
29. Flatz L, Conrad C. Role of T-cell-mediated inflammation in psoriasis: pathogenesis and targeted therapy. Psoriasis (Auckl). 2013;3:1–10. https://doi.org/10.2147/PTT.S26339.
30. Ghoreschi K, Balato A, Enerbäck C, Sabat R. Therapeutics targeting the IL-23 and IL-17 pathway in psoriasis. Lancet. 2021;397(10275):754–66. https://doi.org/10.1016/S0140-6736(21)00184-7.
31. Victor FC, Gottlieb AB. TNF-α and apoptosis: implications for the pathogenesis and treatment of psoriasis. J Drugs Dermatol. 2002;1(3):264–75.
32. Dowlatshahi EA, van der Voort EA, Arends LR, Nijsten T. Markers of systemic inflammation in psoriasis: a systematic review and meta-analysis. Br J Dermatol. 2013;169(2):266–82. https://doi.org/10.1111/bjd.12355.
33. Reddy SP, Shah V V, Lin EJ, Wu JJ. Etanercept. Elsevier; n.d. https://doi.org/10.1016/j.chtm.2016.07.033.
34. Ni C, Reddy SP, Wu JJ. Infliximab. Elsevier; n.d. https://doi.org/10.1016/j.chtm.2016.07.034.
35. Blauvelt A, Chiricozzi A. The immunologic role of IL-17 in psoriasis and psoriatic arthritis pathogenesis. Clin Rev Allergy Immunol. 2018;55(3):379–90. https://doi.org/10.1007/s12016-018-8702-3.
36. Lin EJ, Reddy SP, Shah VV, Wu JJ. Secukinumab. Ther Sev Psoriasis. Elsevier; 2016. p. 139–151. https://doi.org/10.1016/B978-0-323-44797-3.00012-8.
37. Włodarek K, Ponikowska M, Matusiak Ł, Szepietowski JC. Biologics for hidradenitis suppurativa: an update. Immunotherapy. 2019;11(1):45–59. https://doi.org/10.2217/imt-2018-0090.
38. Nia JK, Lebwohl MG. Ustekinumab. Elsevier; n.d. https://doi.org/10.1016/j.chtm.2016.07.036.
39. Blok JL, Li K, Brodmerkel C, Horvátovich P, Jonkman MF, Horváth B. Ustekinumab in hidradenitis suppurativa: clinical results and a search for potential biomarkers in serum. Br J Dermatol. 2016;174(4):839–46. https://doi.org/10.1111/bjd.14338.
40. Min MS, Lebwohl M. Treatment of recalcitrant granuloma annulare (GA) with adalimumab: a single-center, observational study. J Am Acad Dermatol. 2016;74(1):127–33. https://doi.org/10.1016/j.jaad.2015.09.015.
41. Hertl MS, Haendle I, Schuler G, Hertl M. Rapid improvement of recalcitrant disseminated granuloma annulare upon treatment with the tumour necrosis factor-α inhibitor, infliximab. Br J Dermatol. 2005;152(3):552–5. https://doi.org/10.1111/j.1365-2133.2005.06371.x.
42. Murdaca G, Colombo BM, Barabino G, Caiti M, Cagnati P, Puppo F. Anti-tumor necrosis factor-α treatment with infliximab for disseminated granuloma annulare. Am J Clin Dermatol. 2010;11(6):437–9. https://doi.org/10.2165/11311040-000000000-00000.

43. Shupack J, Siu K. Resolving granuloma annulare with etanercept. Arch Dermatol. 2006;142(3):394–5. https://doi.org/10.1001/archderm.142.3.394.
44. Kreuter A, Altmeyer P, Gambichler T. Failure of etanercept therapy in disseminated granuloma annulare. Arch Dermatol. 2006;142(9):1236–7. https://doi.org/10.1001/archderm.142.9.1236.
45. Fayyazi A, Schweyer S, Eichmeyer B, et al. Expression of IF- Ngamma, coexpression of TNFα and matrix metallopro-teinases and apoptosis of T lymphocytes and macrophages in granuloma annulare. Arch Dermatol Res. 2000;292:384–90.
46. Brooklyn TN, Dunnill MG, Shetty A, et al. Infliximab for the treatment of pyoderma gangrenosum: a randomised, double blind, placebo controlled trial. Gut. 2006;55(4):505–9. https://doi.org/10.1136/gut.2005.074815.
47. Goldminz AM, Botto NC, Gottlieb AB. Severely recalcitrant pyoderma gangrenosum successfully treated with ustekinumab. J Am Acad Dermatol. 2012;67(5):e237–8. https://doi.org/10.1016/j.jaad.2012.04.045.
48. Greb JE, Gottlieb AB, Goldminz AM. High-dose ustekinumab for the treatment of severe, recalcitrant pyoderma gangrenosum. Dermatol Ther. 2016;29(6):482–3. https://doi.org/10.1111/dth.12387.
49. Galimberti RL, Vacas AS, Bollea Garlatti ML, Torre AC. The role of interleukin-1β in pyoderma gangrenosum. JAAD Case Rep. 2016;2(5):366–8. Published 2016 Sep 28. https://doi.org/10.1016/j.jdcr.2016.07.007.
50. Tu J, Chan J. Cutaneous sarcoidosis and infliximab: evidence for efficacy in refractory disease. Australas J Dermatol. https://doi.org/10.1111/ajd.12056.
51. Tuchinda P, Bremmer M, Gaspari AA. A case series of refractory cutaneous sarcoidosis successfully treated with infliximab. Dermatol Ther (Heidelb). 2012;2:11.
52. Sené T, Juillard C, Rybojad M, et al. Infliximab as a steroid-sparing agent in refractory cutaneous sarcoidosis: single-center retrospective study of 9 patients. J Am Acad Dermatol. 2012;66:328–32.
53. Heffernan MP, Anadkat MJ. Recalcitrant cutaneous sarcoidosis responding to infliximab. Arch Dermatol. 2005;141:910–1.
54. Meyerle JH, Shorr A. The use of infliximab in cutaneous sarcoidosis. J Drugs Dermatol. 2003;2:413–4.
55. Pariser RJ, Paul J, Hirano S, et al. A double-blind, randomized, placebo controlled trial of adalimumab in the treatment of cutaneous sarcoidosis. J Am Acad Dermatol. 2013;68:765–73.
56. Goel S, Cheema HR, Gillott T, Bhutto H, Quah SA. A case of etanercept (anti-TNF agent) induced granulomas on the lids [published online ahead of print, 2021 Oct 2]. Orbit. 2021;1–3. https://doi.org/10.1080/01676830.2021.1981398.
57. Burns AM, Green PJ, Pasternak S. Etanercept-induced cutaneous and pulmonary sarcoid-like granulomas resolving with adalimumab. J Cutan Pathol. 2012;39(2):289–93. https://doi.org/10.1111/j.1600-0560.2011.01795.x.
58. Daïen CI, Monnier A, Claudepierre P, et al. Sarcoid-like granulomatosis in patients treated with tumor necrosis factor blockers: 10 cases. Rheumatology (Oxford). 2009;48(8):883–6. https://doi.org/10.1093/rheumatology/kep046.
59. Dinarello CA, Simon A, van der Meer JW. Treating inflammation by blocking interleukin-1 in a broad spectrum of diseases. Nat Rev Drug Discov. 2012;11:633–52.
60. Masters SL, Simon A, Aksentijevich I, Kastner DL. Horror autoinflammaticus: the molecular pathophysiology of autoinflammatory disease (*). Annu Rev Immunol. 2009;27:621–68. https://doi.org/10.1146/annurev.immunol.25.022106.141627.
61. Drenth JP, van der Meer JW, Kushner I. Unstimulated peripheral blood mononuclear cells from patients with the hyper-IgD syndrome produce cytokines capable of potent induction of C-reactive protein and serum amyloid A in Hep3B cells. J Immunol. 1996;157:400–4.
62. Martinon F, Burns K, Tschopp J. The inflammasome: a molecular platform triggering activation of inflammatory caspases and processing of proILβ. Mol Cell. 2002;10(2):417–26. https://doi.org/10.1016/s1097-2765(02)00599-3.
63. Zheng D, Liwinski T, Elinav E. Inflammasome activation and regulation: toward a better understanding of complex mechanisms. Cell Discov. 2020;6:36. https://doi.org/10.1038/s41421-020-0167-x.

64. Jensen LE. Targeting the IL-1 family members in skin inflammation. Curr Opin Investig Drugs. 2010;11(11):1211–20.
65. Fenini G, Contassot E, French LE. Potential of IL-1, IL-18 and inflammasome Inhibition for the treatment of inflammatory skin diseases. Front Pharmacol. 2017;8:278. Published 2017 May 22. https://doi.org/10.3389/fphar.2017.00278.

JAK Inhibitors as Immunomodulators

Danielle Peterson, William Damsky, and Brett King

Abstract The dermatologist must focus on the mechanisms of action of the Janus Kinase pathways and the pathogenesis of cytokine production from lymphocytes and transcription of other effector cytokines. The clinical relevance to dermatologists including the impact on inflammation and pathogenesis of diseases such as atopic dermatitis, psoriasis, vitiligo, and other conditions including clinical trial data, topical and systemic therapies, and future medications in development will also be reviewed. A general overview of the efficacy and safety in context to the background behind black box warnings should serve to alleviate concerns for the practicing dermatologist on their incorporation into the therapeutic toolbox.

Keywords Kinase · Auto inflammatory · Antigen · Cytokine · Specificity

Autoimmune, inflammatory, and auto inflammatory diseases—hereafter together called Immune-Mediated Inflammatory Diseases or IMIDs—are diverse, affecting all organs. Cytokines and other mediators secreted from immune cells and other host cells are frequently dysregulated in these diseases. Historically, treatment of these disorders has relied on broad suppression of the immune system. More recently therapeutic antibodies that target specific cytokines or their receptors (biologics) have been developed. Janus kinase (JAK) inhibitors are oral small molecule inhibitors that can also inhibit cytokine signaling by preventing cytokine-induced activation of the downstream JAK-STAT pathway. Here, we review cytokine signaling and the JAK-STAT pathway and discuss their relationship to IMIDs.

D. Peterson · W. Damsky · B. King (✉)
Yale University School of Medicine, New Haven, CT, USA
e-mail: brett.king@yale.edu

N. Bhatia (ed.), *Immunomodulators and Biologics in Dermatologic Treatment*,
https://doi.org/10.1007/978-3-031-66590-5_5

1 IMIDs Pathogenesis

IMIDs are diverse in their presentation, affecting the gut (e.g., inflammatory bowel disease (IBD) including Crohn's disease and ulcerative colitis), the joints (e.g., inflammatory arthritis including rheumatoid arthritis (RA), psoriatic arthritis, etc.), the skin (e.g., atopic dermatitis, alopecia areata, etc.), and other organs. Classically, autoimmune disease was defined as a process mediated primarily by the adaptive immune system (i.e., T and/or B lymphocytes). It is estimated that autoimmune disease affects at least 3–5% of individuals in Western countries, and the incidence has been rising [1–3]. Autoimmunity is largely believed to be the result of complex interactions among host genetics, environmental triggers, and in many cases, likely microbiota [4]. The interplay of these factors ultimately leads to immune responses against self-antigens resulting in tissue damage from inappropriate T and/or B cell activity. Although there are differences in pathogenesis between autoimmune, inflammatory (i.e., atopic dermatitis, asthma, etc.), and auto inflammatory diseases, they have in common dysregulated lymphocyte responses (and cytokine mediated disease, see below). Perhaps the most well-known group of auto inflammatory diseases in dermatology are the "interferonopathies", a group of monogenic disorders relating to dysregulation of viral sensing (Type I interferon) pathways [5]. Type I interferons (IFN-α/β) are central regulators in innate immunity.

As more is learned about IMIDs, neatly grouping diseases into categories is challenging. For instance, considering psoriasis and hidradenitis suppurativa, pathogenesis of both diseases likely involves both innate and adaptive immunity [6–9]. Hence, these and other different diseases are put together under the umbrella IMIDs, with the commonality that all are mediated, at least in part, by cytokines, making them amenable to overlapping treatment approaches.

1.1 Cellular Components of the Immune Response in Autoimmunity

T cells belong to the adaptive immune system and are tasked with identifying foreign peptide antigens and in doing so help to protect against pathogens. During a normal immune response, T cell receptors (TCR) recognize their corresponding antigen in the correct context initiating specific intracellular signaling pathways and activating effector functions. Once the pathogen is eliminated, memory is developed, and the immune response is turned off. However, in autoimmunity, T cells aberrantly react to self or other endogenous antigens resulting in the production of cytokines and other molecules which lead to tissue damage [10, 11]. B cells have varying degrees of involvement in the pathogenesis of different autoimmune diseases through antibody production [12]. Other cell types, including components of the innate immune system (macrophages, neutrophils, natural killer cells, innate lymphoid cells, and others) and other host/stromal cells (keratinocytes, fibroblasts, and endothelial cells) also play role in initiation and/or maintenance of autoimmunity, typically through production of cytokines and other factors.

1.2 Soluble Components of Immune Responses: Cytokines

Several classes of secreted factors regulate immune responses and include cytokines, chemokines, and other molecules. Cytokines are a group of structurally diverse, small, secreted proteins produced by both cells of the immune system as well as other host cells. In general, these molecules coordinate effective immune responses between cells, with most having pro-inflammatory effects, although some have more anti-inflammatory roles (i.e., IL-10, TGF-β). Cytokine signaling occurs when a cytokine that is produced by one cell type binds to specific receptor(s) on target cells, resulting in activation of downstream intracellular signaling pathways and, ultimately, changes in gene expression, which help induce the intended action of the cytokine. Several cytokine families exist and are grouped based on structural similarities of the cytokines and/or their receptors. Some cytokines utilize the Janus kinase (JAK)—signal transducer and activator of transcription (STAT) pathway, while others do not and utilize other conserved pathways such as nuclear-factor kappa B (NF-κB) signaling (Table 1).

Cytokines can function in an autocrine, paracrine and/or endocrine manner. Many cytokines are recognizable because their name is designated as either interleukins

Table 1 Cytokine families and downstream signaling pathways

Cytokines	Family members	Examples of cytokines using these receptors	Downstream pathway	Targeted by JAK inhibitor
IL-1 family	11 cytokines	IL-1α, IL-1β, IL-18	NF-κB	No
TNF family	>17 cytokines	TNF-α, CD40L, FasL	NF-κB	No
4α-helical cytokines	Hematopoietin superfamily Interferons (Type II receptors)	IFN-α/β, IFN-γ, IL-10	JAK-STAT	Yes
4α-helical cytokines	Hematopoetin superfamily Type I receptors*	IL-2, IL-3, IL-4, IL-5, IL-7, IL-9, IL-15, IL-21	JAK-STAT	Yes
Chemokines		CXCL9, CCL2		No
IL-17 family		IL-17	NF-KB	No
Other		TGF-β		No

Listed are major families of cytokines. The downstream pathway(s) activated by each are listed. Some cytokines are JAK-STAT dependent, while others are not

(IL) or interferons (IFN) (i.e. IL-23 or IFN-β); however, not all follow this rule. Other cytokines have names that are descriptive: for example, tumor necrosis factor alpha (TNF-α), oncostatin M (OSM), granulocyte–macrophage colony-stimulating factor (GM-CSF), and even leptin, which is less commonly recognized as having cytokine structure (and also signals via JAK-STAT) [13]. There are over 200 cytokines, [14] and some common examples are included in Table 1. Chemokines, which provide migratory cues to immune cells, [15, 16] are not cytokines and signal via G protein-coupled receptors (GPCRs).

2 Treatment of IMIDs

Historically, treatment of IMIDs has employed relatively non-specific immunosuppressive medications [17]. Such treatment approaches generally act broadly and so may also have significant off-target effects on normal immune function and other homeostatic processes in the body. However, an increased understanding of the pathogenesis of autoimmune diseases has led to the development of a variety of more specific treatment strategies. For, example in many diseases, the use of monoclonal antibodies, which directly inhibit specific cytokines, have revolutionized treatment. Other targeted approaches include small molecule inhibitors of intracellular proteins such as calcineurin inhibitors, and more recently phosphodiesterase inhibitors and JAK inhibitors.

2.1 Conventional Immunosuppressants

This group of medications suppresses immune function broadly by affecting either intracellular receptors (steroids), nucleotide/DNA synthesis (i.e., rapidly proliferating cells) or other intracellular enzymes. Glucocorticoids are the most well-known and, in some ways, most effective group of immunosuppressants.

Antiproliferative agents are a class of steroid-sparing immunosuppressants that are commonly used to treat IMIDs. Included in this class are methotrexate, mycophenolate, azathioprine, and cyclosporine. Methotrexate inhibits the dihydrofolate reductase enzyme, ultimately impairing nucleotide synthesis and thus targeting rapidly proliferating cells, such as T cells (Fig. 1). Mycophenolate and azathioprine have a similar mechanism of action to methotrexate, but target DNA synthesis more specifically in T cells through their inhibition of inosine-5-monophosphate dehydrogenase (IMPDH) and thiopurine methyltransferase (TPMT) enzymes respectively (Fig. 1). Calcineurin inhibitors are another class that include cyclosporine and tacrolimus and work by inhibiting calcineurin which prevents the activation of NFAT, a transcription factor critical for production of pro-inflammatory cytokines by T cells.

Sirolimus and everolimus are mTOR inhibitors. They work by inhibiting the mTORC1 complex, which is a central integrator of cellular growth signals and the

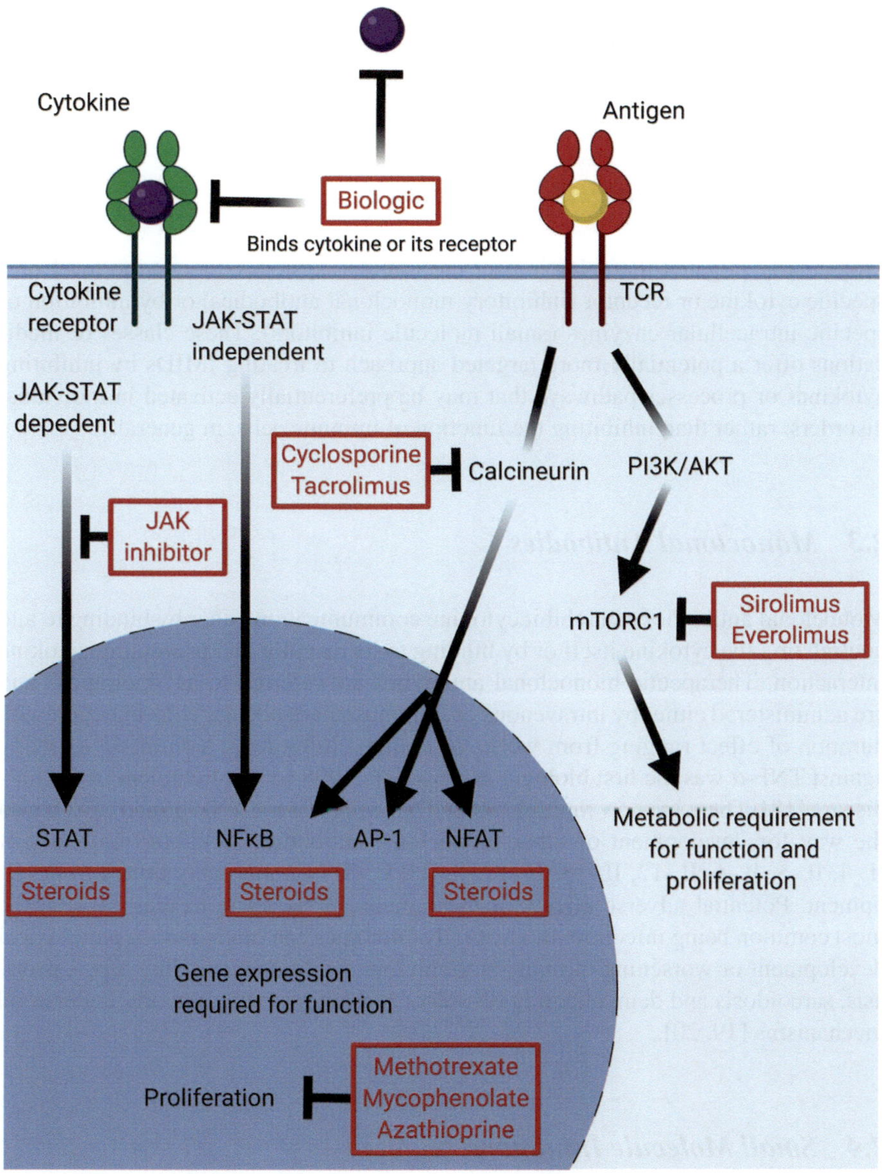

Fig. 1 Molecular targets of medications used to treat autoimmune disease. Monoclonal antibodies (biologics) prevent binding of specific antibodies to their receptors on cells. JAK inhibitors block the downstream effect induced by cytokine – cytokine receptor interactions. mTOR inhibitors block the mTORC1 complex which is activated downstream of the T cell receptor. Calcineurin inhibitors block calcineurin which is activated downstream of the T cell receptor. Corticosteroids have pleiotropic activity and inhibit inflammation at multiple levels. Anti-proliferative agents interfere with DNA synthesis in T cells that is induced by activating signals

metabolic state of immune cells, including T cells; inhibition of mTORC1 can inhibit both T cell function and proliferation. However, mTORC1 is also widely expressed in other cell types where it has a similar function.

2.2 Molecularly Targeted Therapies

Molecularly targeted therapies impact the immune system either at the level of a specific cytokine or receptor (inhibitory monoclonal antibodies) or by inhibition of specific intracellular enzymes (small molecule inhibitors). These classes of medications offer a potentially more targeted approach to treating IMIDs by inhibiting cytokines or processes/pathways that may be preferentially activated in individual disorders, rather than inhibiting the function of immune cells, in general.

2.3 Monoclonal Antibodies

Monoclonal antibodies can inhibit cytokine communication either by binding to and neutralizing the cytokine itself or by binding to its receptor and preventing cytokine interaction. Therapeutic monoclonal antibodies are referred to as "biologics" and are administered either by intravenous or intramuscular/subcutaneous injection with duration of effect ranging from weeks to months. Infliximab, a chimeric antibody against TNF-α was the first biologic approved, in 1998 for the treatment of Crohn's disease [18]. There are now multiple other TNF-α inhibitors. TNF-α inhibitors paved the way for development of other monoclonal antibodies including inhibitors of IL-4, IL-5, IL-6, IL-12, IL-13, IL-17, IL-23, IL-31, among many others in development. Potential adverse effects of these medications relate to their targets; the most common being infection. Interestingly, biologics can rarely induce paradoxical development or worsening of many autoimmune conditions including lupus, psoriasis, sarcoidosis and demyelinating disorders and others through poorly understood mechanisms [19, 20].

2.4 Small Molecule Inhibitors

Newer classes of small molecule inhibitors for treatment of IMIDs inhibit intracellular enzymes and largely fall into a few classes, including phosphodiesterase inhibitors (e.g., roflumilast, apremilast, crisaborole) and JAK inhibitors. Whereas biologics prevent cytokines from binding to their target receptor, small molecule inhibitors block downstream signaling after binding of the cytokine to its receptor. This remainder of this article will focus on JAK-STAT signaling and JAK inhibitors.

3 JAK-STAT Signaling

In order to understand the activity of JAK inhibitors in treating IMIDs, it is important to understand the role of the JAK-STAT pathway (and the cytokines that use it) in normal processes. In the following section we will discuss the JAK-STAT signaling pathway, cytokines that utilize this pathway, and the role of these processes in immunity.

3.1 JAK-STAT Pathway

Cytokine receptors that utilize the JAK-STAT pathway lack their own intrinsic kinase activity and, thus, rely on JAK proteins (which are kinases) for intracellular signaling following cytokine binding. Named after the two-headed mythical Roman god "Janus", Janus kinases are made of pairs of tandem kinase domains and were discovered nearly 30 years ago [21]. There are 4 distinct JAK enzymes in humans: JAK1, JAK2, JAK3 and Tyrosine Kinase 2 (TYK2). JAK3 expression is primarily restricted to immune cells, while JAK1, JAK2, and TYK2 are more widely expressed [22]. JAK protein usage by cytokines has both specificity and redundancy; while there are 4 JAK proteins, which typically act in pairs, there are >50 cytokines that signal through this pathway. For example, IFN-γ signals via the interferon gamma receptor which associates with JAK1 and JAK2, while Type I interferons (IFN-α/β) signal via the interferon alpha receptor which utilizes JAK1 and TYK2. JAK usage by select cytokines is shown in Fig. 2.

Binding of cytokines to their receptors stimulates the dimerization of receptors, leading to JAK phosphorylation and ultimately activation (phosphorylation) of STAT proteins, which dimerize and translocate to the nucleus where they act as transcription factors (Fig. 3). There are 7 STAT proteins: STAT1, STAT2, STAT3, STAT4, STAT5A, STAT5B, and STAT6. Similar to JAKs, there is both specificity and redundancy in STAT usage across cytokines. For example, binding of IL-4 to its receptor results in activation of STAT6 homodimers (via JAK1/JAK3) whereas binding of IL-12 and IL-23 to their receptors results in activation of STAT4 homodimers (via JAK2/TYK2). Additional details of JAK-STAT signaling has been reviewed by others [23].

3.2 Cytokines that Use JAK-STAT

More than 50 cytokines signal via the JAK-STAT pathway and include interleukins, interferons, colony stimulating factors, and others [24–27]. Their broad activity impacts not only inflammation, but also hematopoiesis (erythropoietin, thrombopoietin, granulocyte colony-stimulating factor (G-CSF), and GM-CSF) and non-immune

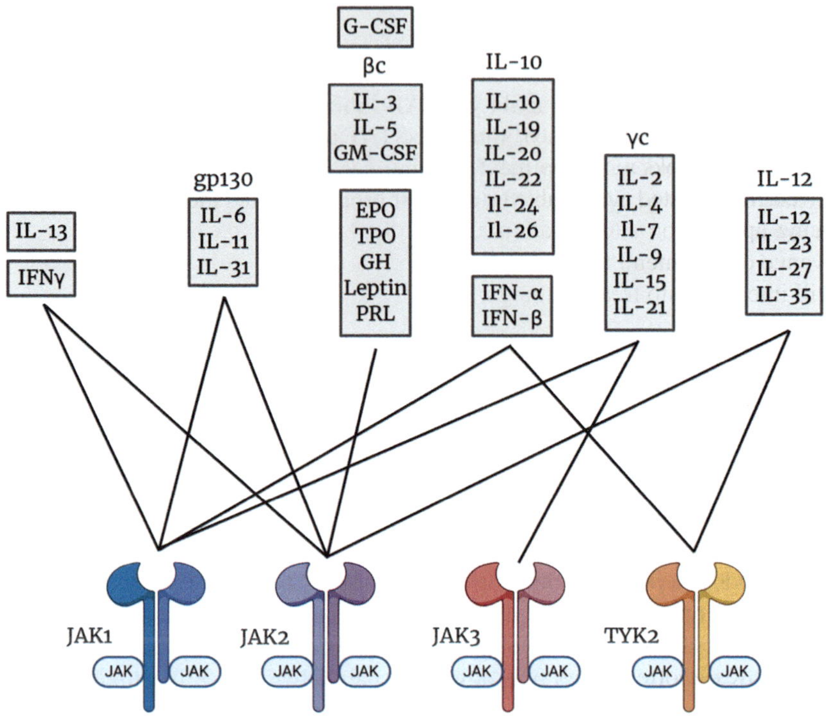

	JAK1	JAK2	JAK3	TYK2
Tofacitinib	15.1	77.4	55.0	489
Ruxolitinib	6.4	8.8	487	30.1
Baricitinib	4	6.6	787	61
Upadacitinib	47	120	2304	4690
Fedratinib	35	1	334	135

Fig. 2 Cytokine and JAK inhibitor specificity for individual JAKs. Various cytokines signal via distinct JAK proteins, as summarized (adapted from Gadina 2018) [26]. The inhibitory concentration IC50 of each of the FDA approved JAK inhibitors is listed; these values are based on enzyme assays. Clinically relevant values have been boxed (i.e. tofacitinib as clinically relevant activity against JAK1, JAK2, and JAK3)

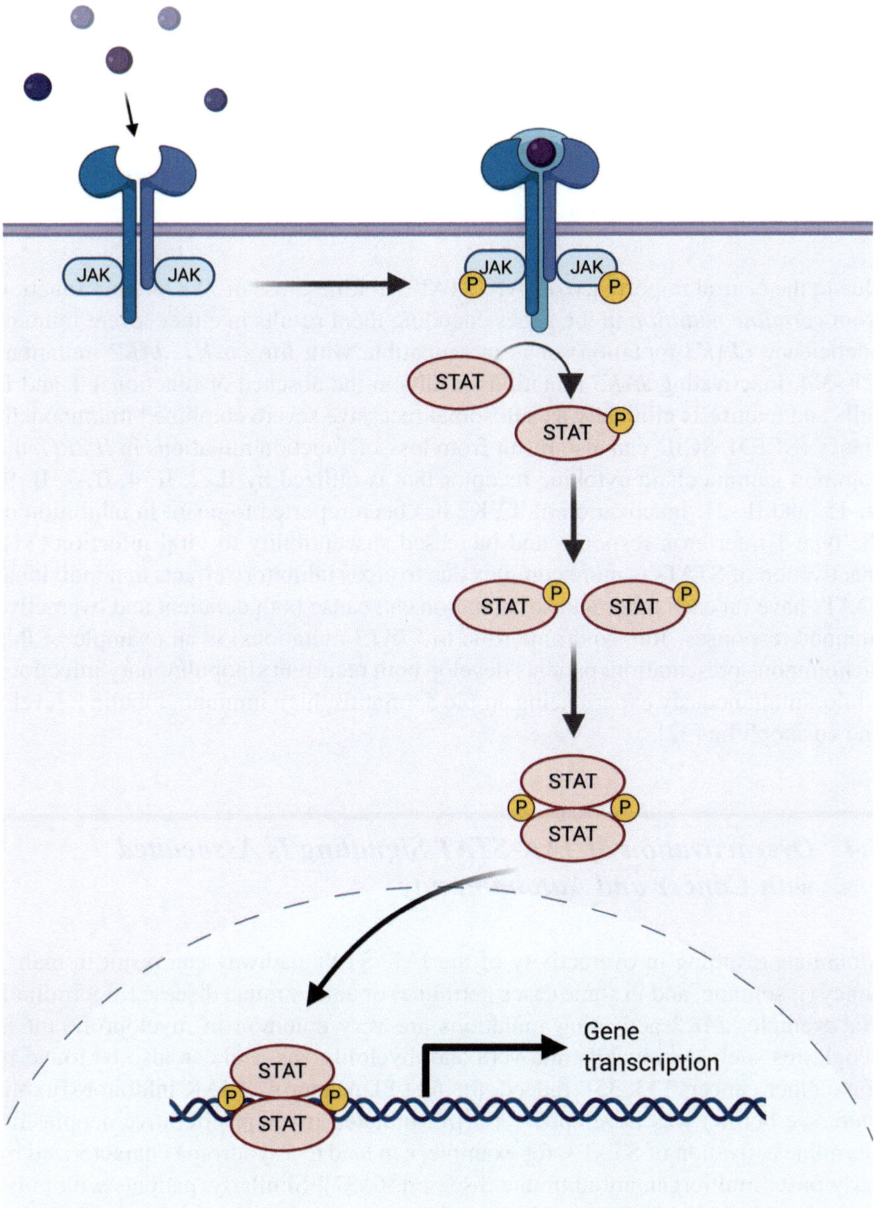

Fig. 3 JAK-STAT signaling. Cytokine binding induces dimerization of the JAK receptors which in turn phosphorylate STAT proteins. STAT proteins then relocate to the nucleus where they act as transcription factors to activate downstream target gene expression

processes (i.e. prolactin, leptin, and growth hormone). Cytokines that use this pathway are summarized in Fig. 2.

3.3 Genetic Inactivation of JAK-STAT Signaling Causes Immunodeficiency

Due to the central importance of JAK-STAT cytokines, loss of JAK protein function from *germline mutation* in the genes encoding them results in either severe immunodeficiency (*JAK3* mutation) or is incompatible with life (*JAK1*, *JAK2* mutation) [28–30]. Inactivating *JAK3* mutations results in the absence of functional T and B cells and manifests clinically as autosomal recessive severe combined immunodeficiency (SCID). SCID can also result from loss-of-function mutations in *IL2RG*, the common gamma chain cytokine receptor that is utilized by IL-2, IL-4, IL-7, IL-9, IL-15, and IL-21. Inactivation of TYK2 has been reported to result in inhibition of the type 1 interferon response and increased susceptibility to viral infection [31]. Inactivation of STATs is more complex due to cross inhibitory effects that individual STATs have on each other and so, mutation can cause both deficient and overactive immune responses. Job syndrome (due to *STAT3* mutations) is an example of this dichotomous presentation; patients develop both recurrent sinopulmonary infectious while simultaneously experiencing atopic dermatitis, high immunoglobulin E levels, and eosinophilia [32].

3.4 Overactivation of JAK-STAT Signaling Is Associated with Cancer and Autoimmunity

Mutations resulting in overactivity of the JAK-STAT pathway can result in malignancy (if somatic, and in some cases germline) or autoimmune disease (if germline). For example, *JAK2* activating mutations are very common in myeloproliferative neoplasms such as polycythemia vera and myelofibrosis, and can also be found in some other cancers [33–35]. Indeed, the first FDA approved JAK inhibitor (ruxolitinib, see below) was developed for *JAK2*-mutated myeloproliferative neoplasms. Germline activation of STAT3, for example, can lead to a syndrome characterized by early onset multiorgan autoimmune disease [36, 37]. Similarly, patients with polymorphisms in JAK-STAT dependent cytokines, cytokine receptors, or even JAK and STAT genes themselves have an increased likelihood of developing specific autoimmune diseases. For example, psoriasis is associated with particular polymorphisms in genes encoding IL-12, IL-23, and TYK2, [7] and IL-4, IL-4 receptor and STAT6 polymorphisms are seen in atopic dermatitis [38]. Strikingly, multiple autoimmune diseases have at least one JAK-STAT related polymorphism described [39].

4 JAK Inhibitors

JAK inhibitors have notable differences and distinguishing properties from biologics.

Due to the redundancy of the JAK-STAT pathway in cytokine signaling, JAK inhibitors inhibit multiple cytokines simultaneously (Fig. 2). If there are multiple cytokine drivers of a disease (e.g., IL-4, IL-13, IL-31, IL-5, and TSLP in atopic dermatitis), then blocking multiple cytokines with a JAK inhibitor may be more efficacious than treatment with a biologic that blocks one or two cytokines. JAK inhibitors are orally administered and have short half-lives. Conceptually, JAK inhibitor selectivity should permit modulation of fewer or larger numbers of cytokines, and so it may be possible to tailor a JAK inhibitor for a specific disease or spectrum of diseases. This, however, may be more complicated than diagrams like Fig. 2 suggest (see *JAK inhibitor specificity* below).

Because JAK inhibitors are small molecules, they can be administered orally or, for some dermatological diseases, topically. When orally administered, they are dosed daily or twice daily. One of the advantages of oral administration is that in the case of an adverse event (e.g., infection) or a patient needing to stop drug temporarily (e.g., a surgical procedure, vaccination, etc.), discontinuation of the JAK inhibitor results in rapid dissipation of effect over hours or days.

4.1 FDA Approved JAK Inhibitors

The first JAK inhibitor, ruxolitinib, was approved in 2011 for myelofibrosis and, in 2012, the second JAK inhibitor, tofacitinib, was approved for RA. Subsequently, ruxolitinib received additional indications in polycythemia vera and graft versus host disease, and tofacitinib for psoriatic arthritis, ulcerative colitis (UC), ankylosing spondylitis and juvenile idiopathic arthritis (in patients ages 2 and older). It was six years after approval of tofacitinib before a third JAK inhibitor, baricitinib, was approved in 2018, again for RA.

There are currently seven JAK inhibitors. In addition to ruxolitinib, tofacitinib, and baricitinib, there are upadacitinib, fedratinib, abrocitinib, and deucravacitinib (Table 2). It is interesting that ruxolitinib, the first approved JAK inhibitor and indicated for myeloproliferative disease, would 10 years later become the first approved JAK inhibitor for dermatological disease, formulated for topical delivery (ruxolitinib 1.5% cream) for treatment of atopic dermatitis and, later, vitiligo. Upadacitinib (originally indicated for RA and then later other inflammatory arthritides and UC) and abrocitinib were the first oral JAK inhibitors approved for treatment of dermatologic disease, in particular atopic dermatitis. Baricitinib was the first JAK inhibitor approved for alopecia areata, an autoimmune form of hair loss. Deucravacitinib is the first approved TYK2 inhibitor and the only JAK inhibitor currently approved for psoriasis.

Table 2 Overview of FDA-approved JAK inhibitors, their indications, dosing and JAK specificity

Variable	Ruxolitinib	Tofacitinib	Baricitinib	Upadacitinib	Abrocitinib	Deucravacitinib
FDA indications	PCV, MF, GVHD	RA, PsA, JIA, UC	RA, AA, AD**	RA, PsA, AS, nr-axSpA, AD, UC, Crohn's	AD	PsO
Dosing	5–25 mg BID	5 mg BID or 11 mg XR QD (RA, PsA) 5–10 mg BID or 11–22 mg XR QD (UC) 3.2–5 mg BID (JIA)	1 mg QD or 2 mg QD (RA) 4 mg QD (RA in Europe and Japan) 2 mg QD or 4 mg QD (AA)	15 mg QD 30 mg QD (AD, nr-axSpA) 45 mg QD for 8–12 weeks (loading dose)	50 mg QD (renal impairment*) 100 mg QD 200 mg QD	6 mg QD
JAK specificity	(IC^{50} values, nM)§					
1	3.3	3.2	5.9	43	29	0.95
2	2.8	4.1	5.7	120	803	>10,000
3	428	1.6	>400	2300	>10,000	>10,000
TYK2	19	34	53	4700	1250	0.2

AA, alopecia areata; *AD, atopic dermatitis*; *AS,* ankylosing spondylitis; *BID*, twice daily; *GVHD,* graft versus host disease; IC_{50}, half-maximal inhibitory concentration; *JIA*, juvenile idiopathic arthritis; *MF*, myelofibrosis; *nr-axSpA*, non-radiographic axial spondyloarthritis; *PCV*, polycythemia vera; *PsA*, psoriatic arthritis; *PsO,* psoriasis; *QD*, once daily; *RA,* rheumatoid arthritis; *UC,* ulcerative colitis; *XR*, extended release

*Estimated glomerular filtration rate (eGFR) 30–59 mL/minute, not recommended in <29 mL/minute

**Baricitinib is approved for AD in Europe, Japan and other parts of the world but not in the US

§ IC50 values measured in cell-free assays and reported to the FDA in New Drug Application for each agent: 202192 (ruxolitinib), 203214 (tofacitinib), 207924 (baricitinib), 211675 (upadacitinib), 213871 (abrocitinib), and 214958 (deucravacitinib)

4.2 *JAK Inhibitor Selectivity/Specificity*

Different JAK inhibitors have selectivity for one or more of the four JAK enzymes. Selectivity is based on IC_{50} values for JAK1, JAK2, JAK3, and TYK2 in cell-free assays. For instance, the IC_{50} values for tofacitinib are 3.2 nM for JAK1, 4.1 nM for JAK2, 1.6 nM for JAK3, and 34 nM for TYK2; based on these values, tofacitinib is sometimes called a JAK1 and JAK3 inhibitor and other times called a pan-JAK inhibitor. Taking account of other considerations, the latter is almost certainly true.

There are several factors that complicate measurement of JAK inhibitor selectivity. One is that IC_{50} values vary between assays. More importantly, selectivity/specificity of small molecules in a cell-free assay may be very different from that in the human body; that is, JAK inhibitor binding and inhibitory behavior may be markedly different in the complex environment of blood and tissue than that measured in a cell-free assay. It is unclear what fold difference in IC_{50} in a cell-free assay is clinically relevant, e.g., tenfold, 100-fold, or 1000-fold? Yet another important consideration are the effects of JAK inhibitors on the broader kinome; that is, different JAK inhibitors may affect other kinases in the kinome.

All of this is to say that characterizing JAK inhibitor "selectivity" or "specificity" is almost certainly overly simplistic and may even be misleading. Ultimately, as the FDA has written, "based on in vitro assays, the relationship between inhibition of specific JAK isoforms and clinical effectiveness is unknown" and, therefore, claims of specificity are not justified and not clinically meaningful.

4.3 JAK Inhibitor Safety: A Boxed Warning

Most JAK inhibitors approved for IMIDs have a boxed warning for malignancy, serious infections, MACE, death, and thrombosis. These warnings emerge from clinical trials of tofacitinib in patients with moderate to severe RA, in particular a post-marketing safety study of patients aged 50 and older with at least one additional cardiovascular risk factor (RA is already a risk factor for MACE). Over a median follow up of 4 years, the risks of malignancy and MACE were 4.2% and 3.4%, respectively, in tofacitinib treated patients compared with 2.9% and 3.4% in adalimumab/etanercept treated patients. The JAK inhibitor deucravacitinib lacks a boxed warning. Because the numbers of adverse events of special interest (those of the boxed warning) in the deucravacitinib trials in psoriasis were not appreciably different from those in other JAK inhibitor trials in other IMIDs, the authors assume that the FDA did not levy the boxed warning on deucravacitinib due to the theoretically narrow spectrum of cytokines inhibited by TYK2 and, thus, an even safer profile.

5 Conclusions

JAK inhibitors are an important class of therapy for IMIDs, with indications across nearly all of medicine, from RA and other forms of inflammatory arthritis to inflammatory bowel disease to atopic dermatitis and other dermatologic diseases; and even myeloproliferative diseases. The broad reach of JAK inhibitors across the spectrum of IMIDs highlights the extraordinary capacity of this class of small molecule inhibitors to achieve immunomodulation in a manner unmatched by any other class of medicine.

References

1. Wang L, Wang F-S, Gershwin ME. Human autoimmune diseases: a comprehensive update. J Intern Med. 2015;278(4):369–95. https://doi.org/10.1111/joim.12395.
2. Cooper GS, St BC. The epidemiology of autoimmune diseases. Autoimmun Rev. 2003;2(3):119–25. https://doi.org/10.1016/S1568-9972(03)00006-5.
3. Bach J-F. The hygiene hypothesis in autoimmunity: the role of pathogens and commensals. Nat Rev Immunol. 2018;18(2):105–20. https://doi.org/10.1038/nri.2017.111.
4. Jörg S, Grohme DA, Erzler M, et al. Environmental factors in autoimmune diseases and their role in multiple sclerosis. Cell Mol Life Sci. 2016;73(24):4611–22. https://doi.org/10.1007/s00018-016-2311-1.
5. Rodero MP, Crow YJ. Type I interferon–mediated monogenic autoinflammation: the type I interferonopathies, a conceptual overview. J Exp Med. 2016;213(12):2527–38. https://doi.org/10.1084/jem.20161596.
6. Tsoi LC, Spain SL, Knight J, et al. Identification of 15 new psoriasis susceptibility loci highlights the role of innate immunity. Nat Genet. 2012;44(12):1341–8. https://doi.org/10.1038/ng.2467.
7. Enerbäck C, Sandin C, Lambert S, et al. The psoriasis-protective TYK2 I684S variant impairs IL-12 stimulated pSTAT4 response in skin-homing CD4+ and CD8+ memory T-cells. Sci Rep. 2018;8(1):7043. https://doi.org/10.1038/s41598-018-25282-2.
8. Zouboulis CC, Nogueira da Costa A, Makrantonaki E, et al. Alterations in innate immunity and epithelial cell differentiation are the molecular pillars of hidradenitis suppurativa. J Eur Acad Dermatology Venereol. 2020;34(4):846–61. https://doi.org/10.1111/jdv.16147.
9. Giamarellos-Bourboulis EJ, Antonopoulou A, Petropoulou C, et al. Altered innate and adaptive immune responses in patients with hidradenitis suppurativa. Br J Dermatol. 2007;156(1):51–6. https://doi.org/10.1111/j.1365-2133.2006.07556.x.
10. Xing L, Dai Z, Jabbari A, et al. Alopecia areata is driven by cytotoxic T lymphocytes and is reversed by JAK inhibition. Nat Med. 2014;20(9):1043–9. https://doi.org/10.1038/nm.3645.
11. Langrish CL, Chen Y, Blumenschein WM, et al. IL-23 drives a pathogenic T cell population that induces autoimmune inflammation. J Exp Med. 2005;201(2):233–40. https://doi.org/10.1084/jem.20041257.
12. Rawlings DJ, Metzler G, Wray-Dutra M, Jackson SW. Altered B cell signalling in autoimmunity. Nat Rev Immunol. 2017;17(7):421–36. https://doi.org/10.1038/nri.2017.24.
13. Holdsworth SR, Gan P-Y. Cytokines: names and numbers you should care about. Clin J Am Soc Nephrol. 2015;10(12):2243–54. https://doi.org/10.2215/CJN.07590714.
14. Proinflammatory cytokines list. Sino Biological. https://www.sinobiological.com/resource/cytokines/all-proinflammatory-cytokines. Accessed 11 June 2020.
15. Griffith JW, Sokol CL, Luster AD. Chemokines and chemokine receptors: positioning cells for host defense and immunity. Annu Rev Immunol. 2014;32(1):659–702. https://doi.org/10.1146/annurev-immunol-032713-120145.
16. Rotondi M, Chiovato L, Romagnani S, Serio M, Romagnani P. Role of chemokines in endocrine autoimmune diseases. Endocr Rev. 2007;28(5):492–520. https://doi.org/10.1210/er.2006-0044.
17. Smilek DE, Ehlers MR, Nepom GT. Restoring the balance: immunotherapeutic combinations for autoimmune disease. Dis Model Mech. 2014;7(5):503–13. https://doi.org/10.1242/dmm.015099.
18. Kornbluth A. Infliximab approved for use in Crohn's disease: a report on the FDA GI advisory committee conference. Inflamm Bowel Dis. 1998;4(4):328–9. https://doi.org/10.1097/00054725-199811000-00014.
19. Ramos-Casals M, Roberto-Perez-Alvarez, Diaz-Lagares C, Cuadrado M-J, Khamashta MA. Autoimmune diseases induced by biological agents. Autoimmun Rev. 2010;9(3):188–93. https://doi.org/10.1016/j.autrev.2009.10.003.
20. Perez-Alvarez R, Pérez-de-Lis M, Ramos-Casals M. Biologics-induced autoimmune diseases. Curr Opin Rheumatol. 2013;25(1):56–64. https://doi.org/10.1097/BOR.0b013e32835b1366.

21. Stark GR, Darnell JE. The JAK-STAT pathway at twenty. Immunity. 2012;36(4):503–14. https://doi.org/10.1016/j.immuni.2012.03.013.
22. Kotyla PJ. Are Janus kinase inhibitors superior over classic biologic agents in RA patients? Biomed Res Int. 2018;2018:7492904. https://doi.org/10.1155/2018/7492904.
23. O'Shea JJ, Plenge R. JAK and STAT signaling molecules in immunoregulation and immune-mediated disease. Immunity. 2012;36(4):542–50. https://doi.org/10.1016/j.immuni.2012.03.014.
24. Gadina M, Le MT, Schwartz DM, et al. Janus kinases to jakinibs: from basic insights to clinical practice. Rheumatology (Oxford). 2019;58(Supplement_1):i4–16. https://doi.org/10.1093/rheumatology/key432.
25. Schwartz DM, Kanno Y, Villarino A, Ward M, Gadina M, O'Shea JJ. JAK inhibition as a therapeutic strategy for immune and inflammatory diseases. Nat Rev Drug Discov. 2017;16(12):843–62. https://doi.org/10.1038/nrd.2017.201.
26. Gadina M, Johnson C, Schwartz D, et al. Translational and clinical advances in JAK-STAT biology: the present and future of jakinibs. J Leukoc Biol. 2018;104(3):499–514. https://doi.org/10.1002/JLB.5RI0218-084R.
27. Villarino AV, Kanno Y, O'Shea JJ. Mechanisms and consequences of Jak-STAT signaling in the immune system. Nat Immunol. 2017;18(4):374–84. https://doi.org/10.1038/ni.3691.
28. Parganas E, Wang D, Stravopodis D, et al. Jak2 is essential for signaling through a variety of cytokine receptors. Cell. 1998;93(3):385–95. https://doi.org/10.1016/s0092-8674(00)81167-8.
29. Neubauer H, Cumano A, Müller M, Wu H, Huffstadt U, Pfeffer K. Jak2 deficiency defines an essential developmental checkpoint in definitive hematopoiesis. Cell. 1998;93(3):397–409. https://doi.org/10.1016/s0092-8674(00)81168-x.
30. Rodig SJ, Meraz MA, White JM, et al. Disruption of the Jak1 gene demonstrates obligatory and nonredundant roles of the Jaks in cytokine-induced biologic responses. Cell. 1998;93(3):373–83. https://doi.org/10.1016/s0092-8674(00)81166-6.
31. Prchal-Murphy M, Semper C, Lassnig C, et al. TYK2 Kinase activity is required for functional type i interferon responses in vivo. Lenz LL, editor. PLoS One. 2012;7(6):e39141. https://doi.org/10.1371/journal.pone.0039141.
32. Zhang Q, Su HC. Hyperimmunoglobulin E syndromes in pediatrics. Curr Opin Pediatr. 2011;23(6):653–8. https://doi.org/10.1097/MOP.0b013e32834c7f65.
33. Baxter EJ, Scott LM, Campbell PJ, et al. Acquired mutation of the tyrosine kinase JAK2 in human myeloproliferative disorders. Lancet (London, England). 365(9464):1054–61. https://doi.org/10.1016/S0140-6736(05)71142-9.
34. James C, Ugo V, Le Couédic J-P, et al. A unique clonal JAK2 mutation leading to constitutive signalling causes polycythaemia vera. Nature. 2005;434(7037):1144–8. https://doi.org/10.1038/nature03546.
35. Kralovics R, Passamonti F, Buser AS, et al. A gain-of-function mutation of JAK2 in myeloproliferative disorders. N Engl J Med. 2005;352(17):1779–90. https://doi.org/10.1056/NEJMoa051113.
36. Milner JD, Vogel TP, Forbes L, et al. Early-onset lymphoproliferation and autoimmunity caused by germline STAT3 gain-of-function mutations. Blood. 2015;125(4):591–9. https://doi.org/10.1182/blood-2014-09-602763.
37. Flanagan SE, Haapaniemi E, Russell MA, et al. Activating germline mutations in STAT3 cause early-onset multi-organ autoimmune disease. Nat Genet. 2014;46(8):812–4. https://doi.org/10.1038/ng.3040.
38. Hershey GKK. IL-13 receptors and signaling pathways: an evolving web. J Allergy Clin Immunol. 2003;111(4):677–90. https://doi.org/10.1067/mai.2003.1333.
39. Banerjee S, Biehl A, Gadina M, Hasni S, Schwartz DM. JAK–STAT signaling as a target for inflammatory and autoimmune diseases: current and future prospects. Drugs. 2017;77(5):521–46. https://doi.org/10.1007/s40265-017-0701-9.

Combinations of Topical and Systemic Immunomodulators

Siamak Moghadam-Kia and Dedee F. Murrell

Abstract Combinations therapies are the cornerstone for many success stories in the treatment of severe autoimmune and inflammatory disorders. Multifaceted approaches to reduce the consequences of steroids as well as the immunosuppressant risks of other aggressive therapies are essential to maintain safety and accomplish remission. At the same time, the clinician has to be aware of the need for regular monitoring of these therapies especially when multidisciplinary care with a rheumatologist or oncologist is part of the plan. The discussion in this chapter will remind the dermatologist that as the captain of the patient's care it is essential to be aware of all of the risks and benefits of immunomodulatory therapies.

Keywords Combinations · Glucocorticoid · Vasculitis · Myopathy · Immunosuppressive

1 Inflammatory Myopathy

The idiopathic inflammatory myopathies (IIMs) are a group of heterogeneous, systemic rheumatic diseases that include adult polymyositis (PM), adult dermatomyositis (DM), myositis associated with other systemic autoimmune rheumatic diseases or cancer, juvenile myositis (juvenile dermatomyositis and juvenile polymyositis), inclusion body myositis (IBM), and necrotizing autoimmune myopathy. The treatment of IIM has been very challenging because of the low incidence and prevalence of these disorders, their variable clinical phenotypes, and the small number of randomized, double-blind clinical trials [1–4]. Traditional treatment approaches include glucocorticoids and conventional immunosuppressive

---

S. Moghadam-Kia
Division of Rheumatology and Clinical Immunology, Department of Medicine, University of Pittsburgh School of Medicine, Pittsburgh, PA, USA
e-mail: moghaddamkias@upmc.edu

D. F. Murrell (✉)
Department of Dermatology, University of New South Wales, Sydney, Australia
e-mail: d.murrell@unsw.edu.au

N. Bhatia (ed.), *Immunomodulators and Biologics in Dermatologic Treatment*,
https://doi.org/10.1007/978-3-031-66590-5_6

or immunomodulatory agents such as methotrexate, azathioprine, mycophenolate mofetil, cyclosporine, tacrolimus, and IVIg. There has been growing interest in assessing novel and targeted therapies such as biologics that target various pathways involved in the pathogenesis of myositis. Biomarkers implicated in the pathogenesis of IIM have been explored using cytokine/chemokine analyses, microarrays and RNA-sequencing analysis, advanced immunohistochemistry, and flow cytometry.

Despite the lack of placebo-controlled clinical trials, glucocorticoids remain the mainstay of initial treatment of IIM. Glucocorticoids are generally initiated with prednisone at a dose of 0.5–1 mg/kg/day in divided doses (generally not exceeding 80 mg daily). After 4 to 6 weeks, the prednisone dose is slowly tapered to the minimum effective dose using the general guideline of a 20–25% drop every month until the daily prednisone dose reaches 5–10 mg/day. The tapering is then frequently stopped while the patient is maintained on ideally 5 mg of prednisone per day for a further 4–6 months depending on the success of the taper, with ideally the total course of steroids being 9–12 months. To taper completely off the 5 mg prednisone, generally what do they do if held at 5 mg for so long. The tapering can be performed faster in patients with no extra-cutaneous manifestations. The first-line conventional immunosuppressive agent for IIM is generally methotrexate or azathioprine.

Methotrexate is a folate antimetabolite that irreversibly bind to and inhibits dihydrofolate reductase, resulting in inhibition of DNA synthesis, repair, and replication. Azathioprine is a derivative of mercaptopurine that inhibits purine metabolism interfering with cellular replication. Hydroxychloroquine can be considered as the initial immunomodulatory therapy for very mild cutaneous dermatomyositis which has better effects on the cutaneous DM [5].

Combinations of topical and systemic immunomodulators can be considered in the initial management of mild or mild to moderate dermatomyositis. **Topical corticosteroids or topical calcineurin inhibitors** are used for local treatment of skin manifestations in dermatomyositis. The first-line topical agent is generally topical glucocorticoid which is typically used for involvement on the scalp, trunk, and extremities to improve the erythema and pruritus associated with DM [6]. High-potency topical glucocorticoids such as clobetasol propionate are typically used to treat the lesions in the locations where the risk of glucocorticoid-induced cutaneous atrophy is low including the dorsum of hands, extensor aspects of elbows and knees, and scalp. Topical clobetasol foam can be helpful for scalp involvement in DM which is often associated with significant pruritus [7]. Lower-potency topical glucocorticoids such as desonide or hydrocortisone can be used for erythema or the heliotrope eruption on the face where the risk of glucocorticoid-induced cutaneous atrophy is higher. Topical calcineurin inhibitors (tacrolimus or pimecrolimus) are generally used for long-term management of skin lesions on the face. Long term topical glucocorticoids on the face should ideally be avoided due to the long term risks on the eyes (cataracts and glaucoma) and skin atrophy. Tacrolimus is a second generation calcineurin inhibitor that binds to an intracellular protein, FKBP-12, resulting in inhibition of T-cell activation. Several case reports and a small, uncontrolled study have suggested efficacy for topical tacrolimus (often tacrolimus 0.1% ointment) in cutaneous dermatomyositis [8]. Potential adverse effects of topical calcineurin inhibitors include burning sensation, exacerbation of pruritus, and in very rare occasions development of internal malignancies. Other therapeutic options for DM-associated pruritus include frequent moisturizing, relaxation techniques, topical menthol lotions, cool compresses, anti-histamines, gabapentin, and pregabalin.

Refractory cutaneous dermatomyositis patients require more aggressive or novel systemic therapies. In a recent analysis of the Rituximab in Myositis trial data, significant improvements were noted in cutaneous disease activity after the addition of rituximab to the standard therapy in adult DM and JDM subjects [9]. In another report, a 32-year-old Japanese patient with an overlap syndrome, including features of DM (proximal muscle weakness, heliotrope rash, and Gottron sign) and systemic sclerosis, inflammatory arthropathy, and CCP positivity (refractory to cyclosporine, IV cyclophosphamide, IVIg, tacrolimus and combination methotrexate and adalimumab) was treated with tocilizumab (anti-IL6 agent) which resulted in resolution of the DM rash and arthritis with gradual improvement in the muscle weakness and CK elevation allowing glucocorticoid tapering [10]. A case of a patient with refractory DM with severe scalp pruritus was treated with apremilast who demonstrated significant improvement in her skin disease and complete resolution of scalp pruritus [11]. In a recent case series including four subjects with refractory DM received Janus kinase inhibition with tofacitinib after failure of several immunosuppressive and immunomodulatory agents which led to significant improvement in cutaneous and extra-cutaneous manifestations [12].

2 Cutaneous Vasculitis

Cutaneous vasculitis is a broad clinical entity. Many forms of systemic vasculitis can affect the skin because of the large number of vessels in the dermis and subcutaneous tissue. Cutaneous vasculitis may be a primary process or may occur secondary to other disease processes such as infection, non-infectious inflammation due to a drug or systemic autoimmune rheumatic disease, and malignancy. Infections and drug reactions are the most common etiologies of cutaneous vasculitis and account for 23 and 20% of cases, respectively. Hepatitis C virus, hepatitis B virus, HIV, cytomegalovirus, parvovirus B19, varicella zoster virus, *Streptococcus spp*, *Staphylococcus aureus*, *Neisseria*, and *Rickettsia* are among the most common infectious causes of cutaneous vasculitis. Penicillins, cephalosporins, sulfonamides, thiazides, allopurinol, phenytoin, tumor necrosis factor (TNF) inhibitors, rituximab, and cocaine are among the most common triggers of drug-induced cutaneous vasculitis. Type II antibody-mediated and type III immune-complex-mediated hypersensitivity are the most common pathogenic mechanisms of cutaneous vasculitis. Urticarial vasculitis may have multiple causes. Cutaneous small vessel vasculitis has been used to refer to vasculitis involving the small blood vessels in the skin including neutrophilic, lymphocytic, and granulomatous vasculitides.

The management of cutaneous small vessel vasculitis involves a workup for potential underlying systemic disorders or an infection that could guide therapy. Topical therapy with glucocorticoid and antibiotic creams may be helpful in some patients, although there is no data to support their use. High-potency topical glucocorticoids such as clobetasol propionate are often used to treat the hands, feet, legs, where the risk of glucocorticoid-induced cutaneous atrophy is low, while lower-potency topical glucocorticoids such as desonide or hydrocortisone are used for disease in areas that are more prone to atrophy, such as face.

Colchicine has been used for cutaneous and articular symptoms. Dapsone has also been used to alleviate cutaneous and articular manifestations. The use of colchicine or dapsone is based on anecdotal studies or small case series. Brief periods of high-dose oral glucocorticoids or immunomodulatory/immunosuppressive agents may be required for severe systemic vasculitis. The immunosuppressive agents usually considered include methotrexate, azathioprine, mycophenolate mofetil, cyclosporine, and cyclophosphamide. Rituximab, TNF inhibitors and omalizumab have shown some efficacy in recent case reports [13–15].

References

1. Oddis CV, Reed AM, Aggarwal R, et al. Rituximab in the treatment of refractory adult and juvenile dermatomyositis and adult polymyositis: a randomized, placebo-phase trial. Arthritis Rheum. 2013;65(2):314–24.
2. Bunch TW, Worthington JW, Combs JJ, Ilstrup DM, Engel AG. Azathioprine with prednisone for polymyositis: a controlled, clinical trial. Ann Intern Med. 1980;92(3):365–9.
3. Dalakas MC, Illa I, Dambrosia JM, et al. A controlled trial of high-dose intravenous immune globulin infusions as treatment for dermatomyositis. N Engl J Med. 1993;329(27):1993–2000.
4. Miller FW, Leitman SF, Cronin ME, et al. Controlled trial of plasma exchange and leukapheresis in polymyositis and dermatomyositis. N Engl J Med. 1992;326(21):1380–4.
5. Pinard J, Femia AN, Roman M, Alsarheed A, Joyce C, Lin J, Vleugels RA. Systemic treatment for clinically amyopathic dermatomyositis at 4 tertiary care centers. JAMA Dermatol. 2019;155(4):494–6.
6. Quain RD, Werth VP. Management of cutaneous dermatomyositis: current therapeutic options. Am J Clin Dermatol. 2006;7(6):341–51.
7. Sontheimer RD. The management of dermatomyositis: current treatment options. Expert Opin Pharmacother. 2004;5(5):1083–99.
8. Hollar CB, Jorizzo JL. Topical tacrolimus 0.1% ointment for refractory skin disease in dermatomyositis: a pilot study. J Dermatolog Treat. 2004;15(1):35–9.
9. Aggarwal R, Loganathan P, Koontz D, Qi Z, Reed AM, Oddis CV. Cutaneous improvement in refractory adult and juvenile dermatomyositis after treatment with rituximab. Rheumatology (Oxford). 2017;56(2):247–54.
10. Kondo M, Murakawa Y, Matsumura T, et al. A case of overlap syndrome successfully treated with tocilizumab: a hopeful treatment strategy for refractory dermatomyositis? Rheumatology (Oxford). 2014;53(10):1907–8.
11. Charlton D, Moghadam-Kia S, Smith K, Aggarwal R, English JC 3rd, Oddis CV. Refractory cutaneous dermatomyositis with severe scalp pruritus responsive to apremilast. J Clin Rheumatol. 2021;27(8S):S561–2.
12. Moghadam-Kia S, Charlton D, Aggarwal R, Oddis CV. Management of refractory cutaneous dermatomyositis: potential role of Janus kinase inhibition with tofacitinib. Rheumatology (Oxford). 2019;58(6):1011–5.
13. Carlson JA, Chen KR. Cutaneous vasculitis update: small vessel neutrophilic vasculitis syndromes. Am J Dermatopathol. 2006;28(6):486–506.

14. Grzeszkiewicz TM, Fiorentino DF. Update on cutaneous vasculitis. Semin Cutan Med Surg. 2006;25(4):221–5.
15. Xu LY, Esparza EM, Anadkat MJ, Crone KG, Brasington RD. Cutaneous manifestations of vasculitis. Semin Arthritis Rheum. 2009;38(5):348–60.
16. de Brito M, Huebner G, Murrell DF, Bullpitt P, Hartmann K. Normocomplementaemic urticarial vasculitis: effective treatment with omalizumab. Clin Transl Allergy. 2018;8:37. https://doi.org/10.1186/s13601-018-0222-y.PMID:30258566;PMCID:PMC6149008.

Nanoparticles as Immunomodulators

Nagasai C. Adusumilli and Adam J. Friedman

Abstract Formulating active ingredients through nanoparticles is increasingly showing promise for a wide range of dermatologic indications. As the mechanistic understanding of nanoparticle interaction with skin strata continues to develop, this strategy of drug formulation and delivery has diverse implications for cutaneous immunomodulation. Nanomedicine may allow localized, topical delivery of both established immunomodulators and novel compounds with anti-inflammatory properties. This brief chapter outlines the principles of nanoformulation for the skin, summarizes the latest evidence for nanoparticles as immunomodulators in dermatology, and discusses future directions for this quickly advancing therapeutic field.

Keywords Nanomedicine · Pharmacokinetics · Immunomodulation · Inflammation · Psoriasis · Cannabinoids · Wound healing

1 Introduction

Nanoparticles, material with a size dimension < 100 nm, are increasingly showing promise across medicine for a wide range of diagnostic applications and treatment indications. Engineered nanoparticles can overcome key physiochemical challenges, opening myriad possibilities for dermatology, such as improved drug delivery methods and formulation of unstable active ingredients for therapeutic effect [1]. Although titanium dioxide and zinc oxide nanoparticles for ultraviolet radiation protection may be the most well-known dermatologic application to date, a growing number of studies are investigating a wide range of active ingredients for their

N. C. Adusumilli
The George Washington University School of Medicine and Health Sciences, Washington, DC, USA

A. J. Friedman (✉)
Department of Dermatology, The George Washington University School of Medicine and Health Sciences, Washington, DC, USA
e-mail: ajfriedman@mfa.gwu.edu

N. Bhatia (ed.), *Immunomodulators and Biologics in Dermatologic Treatment*,
https://doi.org/10.1007/978-3-031-66590-5_7

immunomodulatory properties against inflammatory dermatoses. This chapter will briefly summarize the paradigm for nanoparticle skin penetration, highlight the dermatologic conditions for which nanoparticle immunomodulators show promise, and discuss the likely trends for the future in this rapidly evolving landscape.

2 Skin Penetration with Nanoformulation

For therapeutic use, nanoparticles must penetrate the skin barrier and deliver the active ingredient for the intended molecular interactions in the skin. The drug must penetrate the hydrophobic stratum corneum, with permeation and retention in the more hydrophilic lower layers of the epidermis (Fig. 1). Hair follicles have been shown to be key collection sites for nanoparticles [2, 3]. The varying epidermal thickness and hair follicle density across anatomic locations add to the challenges of topical nanoformulations and comparisons among existing studies.

A wide range of volatile active pharmacological ingredients have been incorporated into nanoparticles, described extensively in preclinical models and clinical trials for various disease states [4–7]. The physiochemical properties of such compounds tend to hinder their utility for medical adoption. High pharmacokinetic variability stems from limitations in stability, solubility, permeation and metabolism. Changes in light and temperature can readily degrade many desired compounds, and rapid permeation and metabolism after systemic and even topical delivery may diminish the intended effects [8].

Upon contact with aqueous solutions, mixtures of solvents, oils, and surfactants can produce nano-sized droplets and stabilize unfavorable pharmacokinetics. Appropriate oil matrices can reduce oxidation and impurities [8], and the dramatic reduction of droplet size augments the surface-to-volume ratio, diffusion, and aqueous solubility [1]. Nanotechnology has successfully encapsulated molecules readily modified by environmental changes and rapid degradation kinetics [4, 7].

When targeting skin-specific cell receptors and limiting topical delivery to the skin, nanoparticles promote the interaction between the lipid matrix and skin strata. Hair follicles have been shown to act as reservoirs of the nanoparticles [2, 3], which diffuse across the epidermis and base of the hair follicle (Fig. 2), releasing the loaded active molecule in a controlled manner [1]. Therefore, despite the vasculature of hair follicles, potential systemic side effects are likely minimized by the controlled release of the nanoparticles, while delivering effective concentrations of the active ingredient.

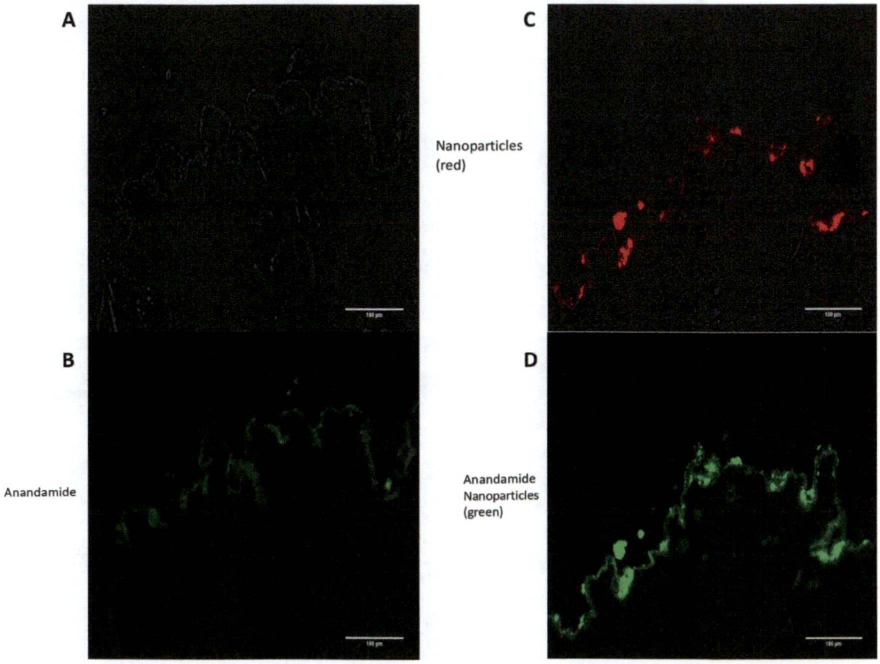

Fig. 1 Epidermal penetration and permeation of nanoparticles loaded with anandamide (AEA), a highly lipophilic endocannabinoid. Epifluorescent histologic images of the skin of MRL/lpr lupus prone mice. (**A**) Phase channel of untreated murine skin. (**B**) Green channel of topically applied AEA mixed with coconut oil vehicle, depicting the inability of the epidermis to retain the control. (**C**) Red channel of topically applied empty nanoparticles, showing penetration of the epidermis and collection in hair follicles. (**D**) Green channel of topically applied nanoparticles loaded with AEA, illustrating the diffusion of the labeled active out from the nanoparticles across the epidermis and deeper at the base of the fair follicles. All scale bars = 100 μm

3 Immunomodulatory Applications in Dermatology

The skin's rich immune system provides both innate and adaptive immune responses to maintain tissue homeostasis. Using nanotechnology to introduce antigens to Langerhans cells and dermal dendritic cells in normal, healthy skin is active area of research for vaccine delivery. Dysregulation of the cascades of cell signalling and cell–cell interactions drives many dermatologic disease states, and nanoparticles loaded with an array of actives demonstrate utility in modulating cutaneous inflammatory processes.

Psoriasis

Improved understanding of the complex, heterogenous pathophysiology of psoriasis has ushered in antibody-based biological treatments for patients. Topical therapy is still crucial for patients with mild disease burden and for maintenance regimens

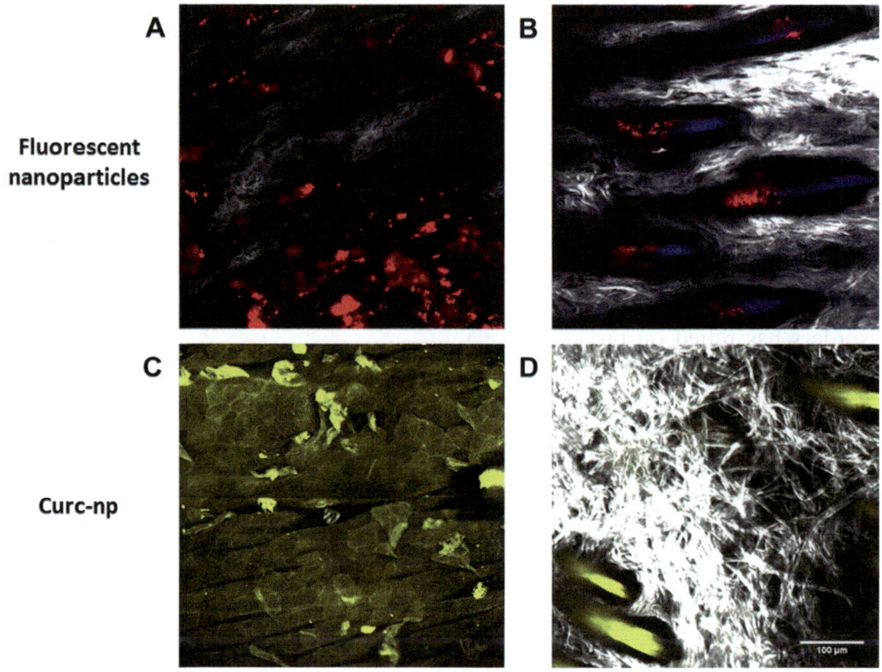

Fig. 2 2-Photon microscopy of nanoparticles topically applied to rat abdomen. (**A**) Image generated 1 h post-application of nanoparticles to the shaved abdomen of a Zucker diabetic fatty rat. Red fluorescently labeled nanoparticles are seen to reside in skin furrows between the white collagen fibers that make up dermal papillae at a depth of 45 mm. (**B**) Image generated 24 h post-application of nanoparticles show residence in hair follicles. Image generated 2 h post-application of curcumin-loaded nanoparticles (curc-np) at 12-mm depth (**C**) and 45 mm depth (**D**); the yellow color is due to the fluorescence of curcumin. From Draganski A, et al. *J Sex Med*. Elsevier Inc. 2018

for patients with moderate to severe forms. As discussed above, nanoformulation can be key in topically delivering treatments safely and effectively. Methotrexate has been a therapeutic workhorse for systemically treating psoriasis, but localized administration to minimize its systemic adverse effects has historically been limited by poor skin penetration. When methotrexate is conjugated with gold nanoparticles (MTX-GNPs), however, topical application mitigates psoriatic skin inflammation in both murine and human xenotransplant models [9, 10]. Visual improvement in the psoriatic phenotype of MTX-GNPs-treated skin was supported by reductions in CD4 + T cells, neutrophils and interleukin (IL)-17 production, without signs of toxicity, such as elevation of serum alanine transaminases. Furthermore, RNA sequencing of psoriatic skin treated with MTX-GNPs shows upregulation of tissue remodelling and wound healing pathways and downregulation of cell proliferation pathways, suggesting that nanoformulated MTX can also modulate stromal mechanisms of disease.

In addition to T cell–mediated dermal inflammation, macrophages drive inflammation in psoriatic plaque via multiple inflammatory signaling pathways, such as nuclear factor kappa B (NF-κB), and subsequent release of pro-inflammatory cytokines and growth factors [11]. In vitro and in human psoriatic plaques, gold nanoparticles (Au-NPs) conditioned with polyphenol-rich extracts specifically and selectively inhibited pro-inflammatory-activated M1 macrophages [12]. Topical treatment of psoriatic plaques with Au-NPs-based ointment reduced the erythema and scaling of psoriatic lesions after 6 weeks of daily application, with decreased CD68-positive infiltrating macrophages and their release of IL-12 and TNF-α [12]. These data suggest that nanoformulated therapies can target epidermal and dermal inflammatory compartments to selectively modulate the dysregulated pathways of psoriasis.

3.1 *Cutaneous Infection and Wound Healing*

Disruption of cutaneous barrier function, seen in prevalent disease states such as diabetes, obesity and atopic dermatitis, increases the risk of microbial invasion and complicates wound healing. Various nanoparticle platforms have been described for inhibiting skin microbes and facilitating the wound healing process. In addition to delivering an active ingredient, several topical nanotechnology systems have intrinsic anti-microbial properties due to the composition of the nanoparticles. Silver nanoparticles' silver ions have been shown to inhibit key bacterial enzymes and induce cell wall and cytoplasmic membrane damage [13]. Chitosan, a crustacean exoskeleton polymer and a unique component of a proprietary nanoparticle platform, disrupts the cell wall and the membrane of microorganisms [14, 15]. Consequently, nanoparticles without any loaded active molecules still exhibit antibacterial effects.

In preclinical studies of wound healing, infection and oxidative stress, curcumin nanoparticles (curc-np) have decreased the in vitro growth of methicillin-resistant *Staphylococcus aureus* (MRSA) and *Pseudomonas aeruginosa* and promoted in vivowound healing of murine burns (Fig. 3) [16–18]. In addition to disrupting the microbes' cellular architecture, curc-np mitigated the zone of inflammation and reduced the mixed inflammatory infiltrate among degenerating and newly formed collagen, accelerating healthy granulation and re-epithelialization. Nitric-oxide-releasing nanoparticles (NO-np) have also been described as highly effective against MRSA in murine models. Nitric oxide (NO) can modulate immune response [19], and topical application is an important therapeutic strategy against superficial skin infections [20, 21]. Nanoencapsulation allows this rapidly metabolized molecule to be delivered in a sustained and controlled manner to wounded, infected skin. Similarly to the curc-np results discussed above, NO-np reduce bacterial burden, decrease suppurative inflammation, and accelerate wound closure [20, 21], likely by limiting inflammatory cascades [22, 23].

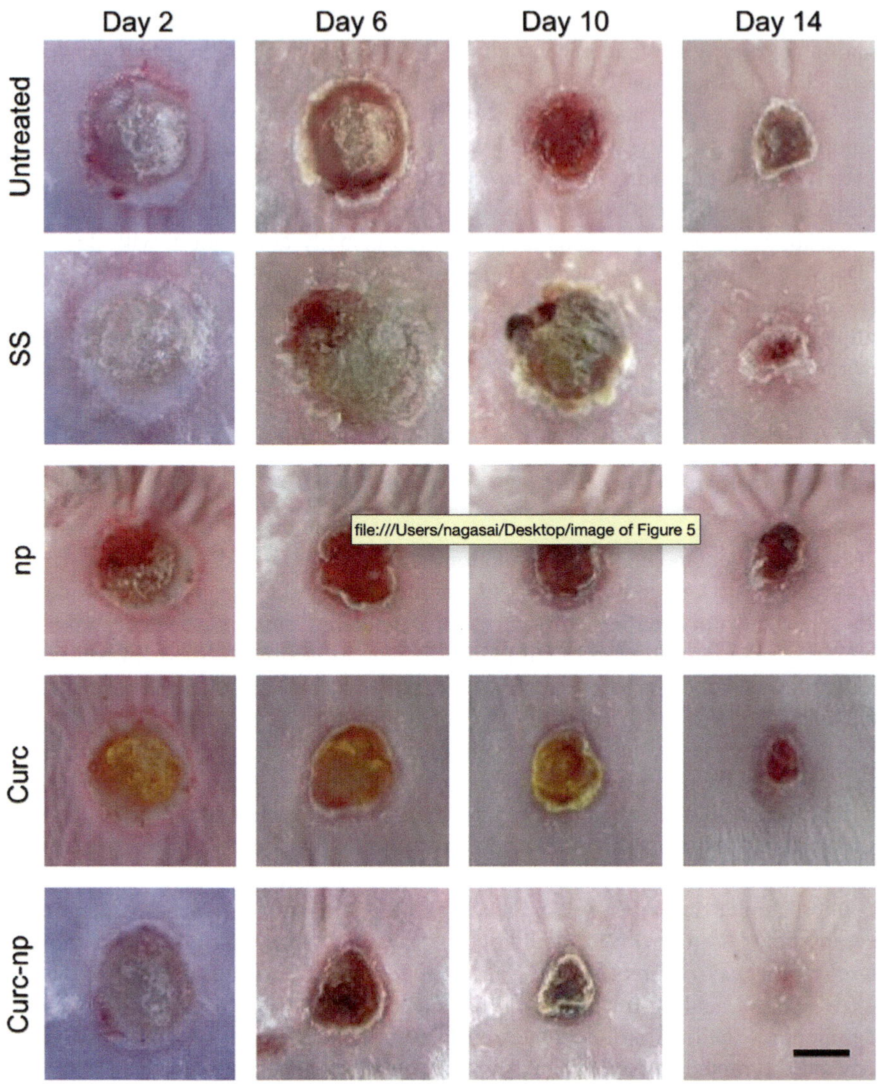

Fig. 3 Curcumin nanoparticles (curc-np) accelerate wound healing in a murine burn model. Representative images of wound healing from days 2–14 in mice treated with curc-np compared to untreated, silver sulfadiazine (SS), coconut oil control (CO), control np (np), and curcumin (curc). Topical administration of curc-np decreased eschar size and qualitatively accelerated healing compared to all other groups. CO (vehicle) control did not differ significantly from untreated control (data not shown). Scale bar = 5 mm. From Krausz AE, et al. *Nanomedicine*. Elsevier Inc. 2015

3.2 *Cutaneous Endocannabinoid System*

The discovery of an intricate endocannabinoid system (ECS) in the skin [24] has spurred the exploration of cannabinoid compounds for dermatological conditions. Although understanding of the molecular mechanisms of cannabinoid activity in inflammatory skin conditions is still nascent [25], cannabinoids demonstrate anti-inflammatory effects against a wide range of dermatologic pathologies, including pruritus, acne vulgaris, asteatotic eczema, and systemic sclerosis cutaneous lupus erythematosus (CLE) [26–29]. Various cutaneous cell populations have CB1 and CB2 receptors and regulatory proteins of the ECS, with translational research models proposing that homeostatic endocannabinoid signalling modulates cutaneous immune processes. G-protein-coupled receptors (GPCR), such as those activated by cannabinoid ligands, actively resolve inflammation rather than allowing a passive dissipation of chemoattractants [30]. Resolvins and protectins, specialized pro-resolving mediators from GPCR activation, cease polymorphonuclear leukocyte infiltration, lessen apoptotic debris, and return inflammatory tissue back to homeostasis [30]. Treatments that manipulate these receptors and regulatory proteins attenuate the inflammatory response induced by Toll-like receptor (TLR)-2, TLR-4 and NF-κB [31–34]. However, cannabinoid-based drugs must penetrate the epidermis and interact with the cutaneous ECS to exert therapeutic benefit.

In a murine model for CLE, topical delivery of 4% arachidonoylethanolamide nanoparticles (AEA-np) significantly improved the skin lesions of MRL/lpr lupus prone mice [35]. The nanoformulation of the highly lipophilic endocannabinoid demonstrated improved CLE Disease Area and Severity Index (CLASI) scores clinically and histologically, likely by downregulating pro-inflammatory cytokines and a hyperactive cell-mediated immune milieu. The immunomodulatory mechanisms of other compounds and disease models may vary and even largely remain unelucidated, but cannabinoids, particularly when formulated to maintain functional integrity and suitable pharmacokinetics, show therapeutic potential through their anti-inflammatory and pro-resolution properties.

4 Future Trends

Therapeutic utility of nanotechnology in dermatology is an active area of investigation. As nanoparticle transport mechanisms in the skin and quantification of nanoparticle dosage, penetration, and therapeutic efficacy are better understood, more applications of nanoparticles for a wide range of immunomodulatory indications are likely. For example, nanoparticles' tropism toward hair follicles suggests potential for inflammatory hair disorders, such as alopecia areata. Severe adverse effects accompany many systemic options, pointing to a need for targeted delivery of immunomodulators such as Janus Kinase inhibitors [36]. Christmann et al. demonstrate proof-of-concept that topically applied nanoparticles do penetrate into human scalp hair follicles, even in the absence of a hair shaft. The ability of hair follicles to serve as a drug depot serves a possible solution to other practical challenges of treating hair loss, such as washing, application frequency, and patient compliance [37].

Nanoparticle accumulation in hair follicles also shows promise in leveraging the abundance of antigen-presenting cells in perifollicular tissue for vaccines. Skin surface stripping can expose hair follicles, and diffused polystyrene nanoparticles are taken up by Langerhans cells and dendritic cells, with subsequent transport to lymph nodes [38, 39]. Separately, multiple microarray patch platforms encapsulated with inactivated influenza antigens propose a transdermal strategy to safely generate antibody levels comparable to intramuscular injection of the vaccine [40, 41]. Although the potential for nanoparticles to induce an intended robust response is promising for vaccine delivery, much more mechanistic understanding is needed to minimize unintentional negative immunological effects, such as contact hypersensitivity.

5 Summary

Nanoformulation is a delivery system well-suited for diverse, novel applications in dermatology. Stratum corneum penetration, epidermal permeation and retention, and follicular collection set up nanoparticles to modulate cutaneous pathophysiology. Proofs of principle are rapidly reported for a multitude of dermatologic contexts, and high-quality clinical trials to establish safety and efficacy are needed to build on this fundamental understanding of therapeutic nanotechnology.

Conflict of Interest The authors have no conflicts of interest to disclose.

References

1. Esposito E, Nastruzzi C, Sguizzato M, Cortesi R. Nanomedicines to treat skin pathologies with natural molecules. Curr Pharm Des. 2019;25(21):2323–37.
2. Draganski A, Tar MT, Villegas G, Friedman JM, Davies KP. Topically applied curcumin-loaded nanoparticles treat erectile dysfunction in a rat model of type-2 diabetes. J Sex Med. 2018;15(5):645–53.
3. Lademann J, Richter H, Schanzer S, et al. Penetration and storage of particles in human skin: perspectives and safety aspects. Eur J Pharm Biopharm. 2011;77(3):465–8.
4. Adusumilli NC, Mordorski B, Nosanchuk J, Friedman JM, Friedman AJ. Curcumin nanoparticles as a photoprotective adjuvant. Exp Dermatol. 2021;30(5):705–9.
5. Krausz AE, Adler BL, Cabral V, Navati M, Doerner J, Charafeddine RA, et al. Curcumin-encapsulated nanoparticles as innovative antimicrobial and wound healing agent. Nanomedicine. 2015;11(1):195–206.
6. Merle P, Blanc JF, Phelip JM, et al. Doxorubicin-loaded nanoparticles for patients with advanced hepatocellular carcinoma after sorafenib treatment failure (RELIVE): a phase 3 randomised controlled trial. Lancet Gastroenterol Hepatol. 2019;4(6):454–65.

7. Friedman AJ, Han G, Navati MS, Chacko M, Gunther L, Alfieri A, et al. Sustained release nitric oxide releasing nanoparticles: characterization of a novel delivery platform based on nitrite containing hydrogel/glass composites. Nitric Oxide. 2008;19(1):12–20.
8. Millar SA, Maguire RF, Yates AS, O'Sullivan SE. Towards better delivery of cannabidiol (CBD). Pharmaceuticals (Basel). 2020;13(9):219.
9. Fratoddi I, Benassi L, Botti E, et al. Effects of topical methotrexate loaded gold nanoparticle in cutaneous inflammatory mouse model. Nanomedicine. 2019;17:276–86.
10. Özcan A, Sahin D, Impellizzieri D, et al. Nanoparticle-coupled topical methotrexate can normalize immune responses and induce tissue remodelling in psoriasis. J Invest Dermatol. 2020;140(5):1003–1014.e8.
11. Ward NL, Loyd CM, Wolfram JA, Diaconu D, Michaels CM, McCormick TS. Depletion of antigen-presenting cells by clodronate liposomes reverses the psoriatic skin phenotype in KC-Tie2 mice. Br J Dermatol. 2011;164(4):750–8.
12. Crisan D, Scharffetter-Kochanek K, Crisan M, et al. Topical silver and gold nanoparticles complexed with Cornus mas suppress inflammation in human psoriasis plaques by inhibiting NF-κB activity. Exp Dermatol. 2018;27(10):1166–9.
13. Chamakura K, Perez-Ballestero R, Luo Z, Bashir S, Liu J. Comparison of bactericidal activities of silver nanoparticles with common chemical disinfectants. Colloids Surf B Biointerfaces. 2011;84(1):88–96.
14. Martinez LR, Han G, Chacko M, Mihu MR, Jacobson M, Gialanella P, et al. Antimicrobial and healing efficacy of sustained release nitric oxide nanoparticles against Staphylococcus aureus skin infection. J Invest Dermatol. 2009;129(10):2463–9.
15. Friedman A, Blecher K, Sanchez D, et al. Susceptibility of Gram-positive and -negative bacteria to novel nitric oxide-releasing nanoparticle technology. Virulence. 2011;2(3):217–21.
16. Liang H, Friedman JM, Nacharaju P. Fabrication of biodegradable PEG-PLA nanospheres for solubility, stabilization, and delivery of curcumin. Artif Cells Nanomed Biotechnol. 2017;45(2):297–304.
17. Krausz AE, Adler BL, Cabral V, et al. Curcumin-encapsulated nanoparticles as innovative antimicrobial and wound healing agent. Nanomedicine. 2015;11(1):195–206.
18. Baltazar LM, Krausz AE, Souza AC, et al. Trichophyton rubrum is inhibited by free and nanoparticle encapsulated curcumin by induction of nitrosative stress after photodynamic activation. PLoS ONE. 2015;10(3): e0120179.
19. Mowbray M, McLintock S, Weerakoon R, et al. Enzyme-independent NO stores in human skin: quantification and influence of UV radiation. J Invest Dermatol. 2009;129(4):834–42.
20. Friedman AJ, Han G, Navati MS, et al. Sustained release nitric oxide releasing nanoparticles: characterization of a novel delivery platform based on nitrite containing hydrogel/glass composites. Nitric Oxide. 2008;19(1):12–20.
21. Martinez LR, Han G, Chacko M, et al. Antimicrobial and healing efficacy of sustained release nitric oxide nanoparticles against Staphylococcus aureus skin infection. J Invest Dermatol. 2009;129(10):2463–9.
22. Navati MS, Lucas A, Liong C, et al. Reducing ischemia/reperfusion Injury by the targeted delivery of nitric oxide from magnetic-field-induced localization of S-nitrosothiol-coated paramagnetic nanoparticles. ACS Appl Bio Mater. 2019;2(7):2907–19.
23. Nacharaju P, Tuckman-Vernon C, Maier KE, et al. A nanoparticle delivery vehicle for S-nitroso-N-acetyl cysteine: sustained vascular response. Nitric Oxide. 2012;27(3):150–60.
24. Kupczyk P, Reich A, Szepietowski JC. Cannabinoid system in the skin—a possible target for future therapies in dermatology. Exp Dermatol. 2009;18(8):669–79.
25. Marks DH, Friedman A. The therapeutic potential of cannabinoids in dermatology. Skin Therapy Lett. 2018;23(6):1–5.
26. Yuan C, Wang XM, Guichard A, et al. N-palmitoylethanolamine and N-acetylethanolamine are effective in asteatotic eczema: Results of a randomized, double-blind, controlled study in 60 patients. Clin Interv Aging. 2014;9:1163–9.
27. Stander S, Reinhardt HW, Luger TA. [Topical cannabinoid agonists. An effective new possibility for treating chronic pruritus]. Hautarzt. 2006;57(9):801–7.

28. Friedman AJ, Momeni K, Kogan M. Topical cannabinoids for the management of psoriasis vulgaris: report of a case and review of the literature. J Drugs Dermatol. 2020;19(8):795.
29. Spiera R, Hummers L, Chung L, et al. Safety and efficacy of lenabasum in a phase ii, randomized, placebo-controlled trial in adults with systemic sclerosis. Arthritis Rheumatol. 2020;72(8):1350–60.
30. Serhan CN. Pro-resolving lipid mediators are leads for resolution physiology. Nature. 2014;510(7503):92–101.
31. Oláh A, Ambrus L, Nicolussi S, et al. Inhibition of fatty acid amide hydrolase exerts cutaneous anti-inflammatory effects both in vitro and in vivo. Exp Dermatol. 2016;25(4):328–30.
32. Oláh A, Markovics A, Szabó-Papp J, et al. Differential effectiveness of selected non-psychotropic phytocannabinoids on human sebocyte functions implicates their introduction in dry/seborrhoeic skin and acne treatment. Exp Dermatol. 2016;25(9):701–7.
33. Gęgotek A, Atalay S, Rogowska-Wrzesińska A, Skrzydlewska E. The effect of cannabidiol on UV-induced changes in intracellular signalling of 3D-cultured skin keratinocytes. Int J Mol Sci. 2021;22(3):1501.
34. Singh A, Singh A, Sand JM, et al. Topically applied Hsp90 inhibitor 17AAG inhibits UVR-induced cutaneous squamous cell carcinomas. J Invest Dermatol. 2015;135(4):1098–107.
35. Chalmers S, Garcia S, Draganski A, Doerner J, Friedman A, Friedman J, Putterman C. Topical endocannabinoid administration protects MRL-Lpr/Lpr mice from cutaneous lupus erythematosus [abstract]. Arthritis Rheumatol. 2018;70(suppl 10).
36. Xing L, Dai Z, Jabbari A, et al. Alopecia areata is driven by cytotoxic T lymphocytes and is reversed by JAK inhibition. Nat Med. 2014;20(9):1043–9.
37. Christmann R, Thomas C, Jager N, et al. Nanoparticle targeting to scalp hair follicles: new perspectives for a topical therapy for alopecia areata. J Invest Dermatol. 2020;140(1):243-246.e5.
38. Vogt A, Hadam S, Deckert I, et al. Hair follicle targeting, penetration enhancement and Langerhans cell activation make cyanoacrylate skin surface stripping a promising delivery technique for transcutaneous immunization with large molecules and particle-based vaccines. Exp Dermatol. 2015;24(1):73–5.
39. Mahe B, Vogt A, Liard C, et al. Nanoparticle-based targeting of vaccine compounds to skin antigen-presenting cells by hair follicles and their transport in mice. J Invest Dermatol. 2009;129(5):1156–64.
40. Rouphael NG, Paine M, Mosley R, et al; TIV-MNP 2015 Study Group. The safety, immunogenicity, and acceptability of inactivated influenza vaccine delivered by microneedle patch (TIV-MNP 2015): a randomised, partly blinded, placebo-controlled, phase 1 trial. Lancet. 2017;390(10095):649–58.
41. Fernando GJP, Hickling J, Jayashi Flores CM, et al. Safety, tolerability, acceptability and immunogenicity of an influenza vaccine delivered to human skin by a novel high-density microprojection array patch (Nanopatch™). Vaccine. 2018;36(26):3779–88.

Antibiotics and Antimicrobials as Immunomodulators

Divya Chopra, Neil Seth, Scott A. Elman, and Hadar Lev-Tov

Abstract Infectious processes are by nature immunomodulators through their effect on their host. Antimicrobial agents are drugs designed primarily to directly kill pathogens or to inhibit their reproduction or growth. However, many of these agents have additional immunomodulatory effects, direct and indirect, due to common pathways and structural similarities between pathogens and humans. Dermatologists are amongst the top prescribers of antimicrobial agents and often utilize antimicrobials for their immunomodulatory actions. This chapter will review the immunomodulatory effects of antibiotics, antifungal, and antiparasitic agents as well their current uses in dermatology.

Keywords Antibiotics · Antifungal · Antiparasitic · Cytokine · Chemotaxis · Immunomodulation · Anti-inflammatory

1 Introduction

Microbial infections are potent immunomodulators that stimulate significant changes in their host's homeostatic mechanisms [1]. Antimicrobials, including antibiotics, antivirals, and antiparasitics, are important agents that treat infections by directly reducing the number of pathologic agents or altering the mechanisms that allow their infectious capabilities. However, microbes and humans share many "essentials of life" including similar biochemical pathways, genetic structures, and energy sources like adenosine triphosphate [2]. Recently, antimicrobials have been recognized for their effect on modulating the immune system of hosts independently from their effect on microbes.

Antimicrobials are a keystone of treatment for dermatologists. Dermatologists prescribe more antibiotics per provider than any other specialty [3]. Besides cutaneous infections, dermatologists commonly prescribe antibiotics for treatment of

D. Chopra · N. Seth · S. A. Elman · H. Lev-Tov (✉)
Dr. Phillip Frost Department of Dermatology and Cutaneous Surgery, University of Miami Miller School of Medicine, Miami, USA
e-mail: hlevtov@med.miami.edu

N. Bhatia (ed.), *Immunomodulators and Biologics in Dermatologic Treatment*,
https://doi.org/10.1007/978-3-031-66590-5_8

noninfectious inflammatory diseases. This chapter will explore how antimicrobials are used as immunomodulators to treat dermatologic conditions (Table 1).

Table 1 Summary of antimicrobial drugs, their mechanism of action and use in clinical dermatology

Class	Mechanism of action	Disease
Antibacterials		
Clindamycin	Inhibit proinflammatory cytokines (IL-1α, TNF-α) Modulate cytokine production in LPS-stimulated macrophages Suppress chemotaxis of neutrophils	Acne Hidradenitis suppurativa Rosacea
Clofazimine	Decrease neutrophil mobility Inhibit activation and proliferation of T lymphocytes	Pyoderma gangrenosum Granuloma faciale
Dapsone	Antineutrophil activity Inhibits prostaglandins and leukotrienes	Acne Pyoderma gangrenosum Behcet's Disease Lichen planus Bullous pemphigoid
Macrolides	Inhibit production of proinflammatory cytokines (IL-1, IL-6, IL-8, TNF-a) Increase production of anti-inflammatory cytokines (IL-4, IL-10) Inhibit neutrophil chemotaxis	Psoriasis Rosacea Pityriasis rosea Pityriasis lichenoides
Metronidazole	Inhibit free radical generation by neutrophils and oxidative damage	Acne Rosacea Seborrheic dermatitis
Rifampicin	Inhibit neutrophil chemotaxis and function Inhibit T-lymphocyte function Inhibit proinflammatory cytokines (IL-1α, TNF-α) Increase production of anti-inflammatory cytokines (IL-6, IL-10)	Hidradenitis suppurativa Psoriasis Pruritus secondary to primary biliary cholangitis
Tetracyclines	Inhibit neutrophil chemotaxis and function Inhibit proinflammatory cytokines (IL-1α, TNF-α, IL-8) Inhibit T-lymphocyte proliferation and response Inhibit MMPs and mast cell activation	Acne Immunobullous diseases Lichen planus Rosacea Pyoderma gangrenosum

(continued)

Table 1 (continued)

Class	Mechanism of action	Disease
Antifungals		
Azoles	Inhibit proinflammatory cytokines (IL-8, 5-LO) Inhibit neutrophil chemotaxis Inhibit T-lymphocyte proliferation and response Antiangiogenic Anti-malignancy	Seborrheic dermatitis Palmoplantar pustulosis Lichen planus Infantile hemangioma Basal cell carcinoma
Antiparasitics		
Chloroquine and Hydroxychloroquine	Inhibit proinflammatory cytokines (IL-1α, TNF-α, IFN-γ) Endosomal inhibition of toll-like receptor Inhibit prostaglandin activity, leukotriene synthesis, and histamine release Impaired chemotaxis, phagocytosis, and superoxide production by neutrophils	Systemic lupus erythematous Granulomatous disorders Lichen planus Urticaria
Levamisole*	Immunostimulatory of T-lymphocyte function Increase production of anti-inflammatory cytokines (IL-2,IL-12) Inhibit neutrophil chemotaxis	Acne Systemic lupus erythematous Vitiligo
Ivermectin	Inhibit neutrophil chemotaxis Inhibit proinflammatory cytokines (IL-1α, TNF-α) Increase production of anti-inflammatory cytokines (IL-23)	Rosacea

*Levamisole has been withdrawn from the market in the United States

2 Antibiotics

2.1 Clindamycin

Clindamycin is a synthetic derivative of lincomycin, an antibiotic derived from the bacteria *Streptomyces lincolnensis*. It is a bacteriostatic agent that exerts its effect by binding irreversibly to the 50 s ribosomal subunit and inhibiting intracellular protein synthesis. Clindamycin can be administered in intravenous, oral, and topical formulations. In its oral form, it is rapidly absorbed with up to 90% oral bioavailability [4]. In several studies, topical application of clindamycin demonstrated small amounts of systemic absorption, approximately 4–5% [5, 6]. Clindamycin is most effective against Gram-positive cocci, specifically methicillin-resistant *Staphylococcus aureus*, and both Gram-positive and -negative anaerobes.

Clindamycin produces immunomodulatory effects that aid in the treatment of numerous dermatological conditions. For instance, in the treatment of acne vulgaris and rosacea, clindamycin has been shown to modulate cytokine production in lipopolysaccharide (LPS)-stimulated macrophages as well as decrease the production of pro-inflammatory cytokines like tumor necrosis factor (TNF)-α, interleukin (IL)-1, and IL-6 [7]. Furthermore, hidradenitis suppurativa is a disease of the pilosebaceous unit that is commonly treated with clindamycin. Use of clindamycin suppresses complement-derived chemotaxis of neutrophils to reduce inflammation [2, 8]. Additionally, clindamycin has been predicted to enhance the uptake of microorganisms by phagocytic cells in the host [2].

2.2 Clofazimine

Clofazimine is a riminophenazine antibiotic known for its antimycobacterial properties, specifically multidrug resistant *Mycobacterium tuberculosis.* Its exact mechanism of action is unknown although proposed mechanisms include intracellular redox cycling and membrane destabilization and dysfunction. It is a highly lipophilic drug and concentrates in fatty tissues as well as cells of the mononuclear phagocyte system [9].

Clofazimine exerts its immunomodulatory effect primarily through inhibiting activation and proliferation of T lymphocytes. This is effected through dysfunction of potassium channels, decreased sodium-phosphate ATPase activity, and increased release of reactive oxygen species and E-series prostaglandins (PGE), especially PGE-2, by neutrophils and monocytes [9]. Clofazimine's inhibitory effect on neutrophil motility and lymphocyte transformation is efficacious in treating pyoderma gangrenosum, granulomatous cheilitis, granuloma faciale, and lupus miliaris disseminatus facei.

2.3 Dapsone

Dapsone is an aniline derivative from a group of synthetic sulfones. It is a bacteriostatic agent that inhibits synthesis of dihydrofolic acid and therefore nucleic acid synthesis. Dapsone is easily and rapidly absorbed in the gastrointestinal tract, reaching bioavailability of over 86% [10]. Once it is metabolized by the liver through acetylation and hydroxylation, a derivative molecule known as dapsone hydroxylamine (DDS-NOH) is generated through a metabolic pathway similar to that in lesional skin of inflammatory dermatoses meditated by activated neutrophils.

Dapsone generates an anti-inflammatory effect similar that of classic non-steroidal anti-inflammatory agents such as ibuprofen. It suppresses both intra- and extracellular production of superoxide by inhibiting calcium influx channels. This in turn prevents degranulation of neutrophils. Dapsone also exhibits immunomodulatory effects on neutrophils through alteration of chemotaxis, cellular adhesion molecule dysfunction, decreased prostaglandin and leukotriene synthesis, and inhibition of IL-8. As such, dapsone is an effective agent at treating inflammatory dermatoses mediated through neutrophils such as Bechet's disease, pyoderma gangrenosum, bullous disorders, and vasculitides. Currently, dapsone is only FDA-approved for use in leprosy, dermatitis herpetiformis, and acne vulgaris [10, 11].

2.4 Macrolides

Macrolides, including azithromycin, erythromycin, clarithromycin, and roxithromycin are a large group of antibiotics that contain a large macrocyclic lactone ring structure. They are bacteriostatic agents that bind irreversibly to the bacterial 50 s ribosomal subunit to halt bacterial protein synthesis. Because the 50 s subunit structure is widely conserved amongst bacteria, macrolides have a broad spectrum of effect including Gram-positive bacteria and some Gram-negative species including intracellular microbes.

The immunomodulatory effect of macrolides was first observed in hypersecretory pulmonary conditions like cystic fibrosis and diffuse panbronchiolitis. This effect was thought to work on several different targets in the host immune response. Macrolides were found to suppress neutrophil chemotaxis. Neutrophil extravasation to tissue is decreased by macrolide-induced dysfunction of adhesion molecules. Macrolides were also found to inhibit production of proinflammatory cytokines such as IL-1, IL-6, IL-8, and TNF-α while increasing production of IL-4 and IL-10 [12, 13].

These effects extend to inflammatory dermatoses. In rosacea, azithromycin is an efficacious treatment through its inhibition of proinflammatory cytokines. Similarly, psoriasis is an inflammatory condition characterized by overproduction of proinflammatory cytokines and neutrophils. In psoriasis, any drug in the macrolide class is potentially efficacious in treating pruritic symptoms and decreasing severity of disease as seen by a decrease in psoriasis area severity index (PASI) of treated induviduals [14, 15]. Despite the challenge of evaluating any treatment for a self-resolving disease, a trial investigating the treatment of people with pityriasis rosea with erythromycin resulted in complete response in 73% of the participants [16]. However, treatment with azithromycin was did not achieve similar results [16, 17]. Similar results of treatment with erythromycin were seen in pityriasis lichenoides [18, 19].

2.5 Metronidazole

Metronidazole belongs to the nitroimidazole class. It is a bactericidal agent that acts by forming nitroso radicals to disrupt nucleic acid synthesis and disrupt DNA of microbial cells. The antibiotic must first be reduced to be active which occurs only with anaerobic bacteria and protozoan, leaving it ineffective against aerobic bacteria [20]. Metronidazole demonstrates a concentration-dependent bactericidal effect, extended half-life, and prolonged activity at higher doses [21].

Metronidazole exerts its anti-inflammatory effects through inhibition of free radical generation by neutrophils and oxidative tissue damage [22]. This anti-inflammatory action contributes to the efficacy of topical metronidazole in treatment of acne and rosacea. In a study on rosacea, application of topical metronidazole was found to improve inflammatory lesions up to 96% [23]. Topical metronidazole was also found to lead to marked improvement up to complete clearance of disease in seborrheic dermatitis [24, 25].

2.6 Rifampicin

Rifampicin is a semisynthetic macrocyclic antibiotic belonging to the rifamycin class. It has bactericidal activity through inhibition of DNA-dependent RNA polymerase whether by sterically blocking the elongating RNA chain or by decreasing affinity of RNA polymerase for elongating RNA chains. Rifampicin is absorbed in the gastrointestinal tract and then hydrolyzed in bile.

Rifampicin as well as other drugs from the rifamycin class exert an anti-inflammatory effect through inhibition of human neutrophil function and T-cell function. These drugs carry an acidic substituent at C3 which decreases superoxide generation. They have also been shown to suppress chemotaxis of neutrophils [26]. Additionally, rifampicin decreases production of proinflammatory cytokines such as IL-1α and TNF-α whereas it increases production of IL-6 and IL-10 [27].

Hidradenitis suppurativa responds well to combination therapy of clindamycin and rifampicin likely due to their additive anti-inflammatory effect [28]. Psoriasis also responds well to the immunosuppressive properties of rifampicin. One clinical trial asserts that rifampicin similarly affected psoriasis patients with and without concomitant bacterial infection suggesting that the effect was not solely dependent on its antimicrobial properties [29, 30]. In the case of cholestatic itch resulting from primary biliary cholangitis, rifampin upregulates cytochrome P3A to promote metabolism of endogenous pruritogenic compounds and competes for uptake of bile salts into hepatocytes [31].

2.7 Tetracyclines

Tetracyclines are a family of broad-spectrum antibiotics including tetracycline, doxycycline, minocycline, and lymecycline. Each has a basic structure composed of four fused rings. They are bacteriostatic agents that prevent binding of aminoacyl-tRNA to the bacterial 30 s ribosomal subunit to inhibit protein synthesis. They exhibit effects on gram-positive and -negative bacteria as well as atypical microbes such as mycoplasmas and rickettsiae.

Many tetracyclines have anti-inflammatory properties. Notably, tetracycline, doxycycline, and minocycline, when used at sub-antimicrobial dosing decrease neutrophil chemotaxis through decreased production of cytokines like peptide chemotaxis factor and lipase [32]. Additionally, doxycycline inhibits the production of proinflammatory cytokines such as IL-1α, IL-6, and TNF-α [33]. Tetracyclines inhibit leukocyte migration through chelation of intracellular calcium necessary for microtubule assembly that allow for cellular movement [34, 35]. Similarly, tetracyclines chelate zinc needed for matrix metalloproteinases (MMPs) function [36]. Tetracyclines, specifically minocycline, demonstrate antioxidant properties as well [37]. An inhibitory effect of tetracyclines on granulomas has been observed but the exact mechanism is unknown. One proposed theory is the inhibition of protein kinase C [38].

Rosacea is frequently treated with doxycycline and minocycline. Immunomodulatory mechanisms of action proposed include inhibited leukocyte migration, inhibited neutrophil activation, reduced pro-inflammatory cytokines, and reduced vasodilation through an inhibitory effect on MMP-9, nitrous oxide (NO), and vascular endothelial growth factor (VEGF) [39]. Sub-antimicrobial dosing of doxycycline was found to be more efficacious in treatment of rosacea when compared to antimicrobial dosing and placebo [40]. A similar statistical effect was not seen in the treatment of acne, however, the use of sub-antimicrobial dosing demonstrated equivalent improvement with less adverse effects reported [41]. The immunomodulatory effect is likely similar in acne and rosacea however, acne patients tend to have higher levels of reactive oxygen species suggesting that tetracycline's antioxidant effects play a larger role in the overall anti-inflammatory effect of the treatment in acne [35].

The ability of tetracyclines to inhibit T-cell activation, neutrophil dysfunction, and generally decrease other proinflammatory processes (e.g. MMPs inhibition) is leveraged in the treatment of a wide variety of dermatoses. People with lichen planopilaris respond well to treatment with tetracycline and doxycycline likely due to the inhibition of T-cell response [42]. Autoimmune bullous disorders such as cicatricial pemphigoid and linear IgA bullous dermatosis respond well to treatment with tetracyclines and demonstrate decreased erythema and skin blistering which are likely mediated by inhibition of MMPs production and mast cell activation [35]. The positive therapeutic effect of doxycycline and minocycline on neutrophilic dermatoses, such as pyoderma gangrenosum and Sweet's syndrome, is the result of decreased neutrophil chemotaxis and degranulation [43, 44].

3 Antifungals

3.1 Azoles

Azoles are a broad class of antifungal agents that are divided into two subclasses: (1) imidazole which contain two nitrogen atoms in a five-member aromatic ring and (2) triazoles which contain three nitrogen atoms. Both classes ultimately act by inhibiting 14-alpha-demethylase which is a cytochrome P450 (CYP) enzyme. 14-alpha-demethylase synthesizes ergosterol which is an essential component of the fungal cell membrane. By inhibiting this key enzyme, azoles exhibit fungistatic activity by disrupting the cell function and growth. High dosages of some agents in the azole class such as ketoconazole exhibit toxicity due to its affinity to human CYP enzymes [45].

Few azole agents such as ketoconazole and itraconazole demonstrate anti-inflammatory effects. Azoles can inhibit the formation of pro-inflammatory cytokines such as 5- lipoxygenase, the production of IL-8, and neutrophil chemotaxis. Topical application of ketoconazole was shown to be superior to control in inhibiting UVB-induced erythema. It was also superior to econazole, another azole, and hydrocortisone [46]. These effects can be especially beneficial in treating seborrheic dermatitis [47]. Yeasts of the *Malassezia* genus can be a source of inflammatory reactions in patients with seborrheic dermatitis. In a randomized, double-blind study, ketoconazole 2% gel was significantly more efficacious in treating seborrheic dermatitis when compared to a control vehicle gel [48]. While the antifungal action of ketoconazole cannot be discounted, the anti-inflammatory effects is likely complementary helps to limit irritation and restore the barrier function [49, 50].

The immunomodulatory effect of itraconazole has been documented as well [51]. The inhibitory effect on neutrophils and pro-inflammatory cytokines is a possible mechanism of itraconazole treatment. Two studies of investigating the treatment of palmoplantar pustulosis with itraconazole demonstrated significant reduction of pustules formation, desquamation, and erythema with maintenance dosing [52, 53]. The efficacy of pulsed itraconazole treatment for lichen planus was demonstrated in a prospective study. Itraconazole treatment resulted in decreased lesion count and pruritis [54]. The effect of itraconazole on lichen planus can also be attributed to its ability to suppress T-lymphocyte proliferation in-vitro [55]. This immunomodulatory effect of itraconazole is hypothesized to play a role in treatment of mycosis fungoides. One case study reported complete resolution of lesions in one week after treatment with two hundred milligrams of itraconazole per day in biopsy-confirmed plaque stage mycosis fungoides with multiple negative skin scrapings [56].

Interestingly, itraconazole has been demonstrated to inhibit the Hedgehog (Hh) pathway and cancer growth by inhibiting activation of the Smoothened (SMO) receptor. Activation of the Hh pathway via SMO is an established cause for cutaneous malignancy, namely basal cell carcinoma (BCC) [57]. One cohort study demonstrated decreased cell proliferation and tumor area in BCC with use of itraconazole [58]. There is some evidence that the Hh pathway can be proangiogenic. Inhibition of this pathway as well as itraconazole's inhibitory effect on the mTOR pathway may explain its antiangiogenic effect which is useful in treating infantile hemangioma [59, 60]. One comparative analysis of itraconazole to propranolol, a β-blocker, exhibited comparable efficacy and safety profiles [61].

4 Antiparasitics

4.1 Antimalarials

Quinine and its derivatives are a class of antimalarials commonly used in treatment of various dermatologic and autoimmune disorders. Quinine is a naturally occurring alkaloid first discovered in 1820. Its first use in dermatology was to treat discoid lupus erythematous in 1894. Its derivates, chloroquine (CQ) and hydroxychloroquine (HCQ), were synthesized about a century later and were initially designed for the prophylactic treatment of malaria. The quinine class interfere with lysosomal activity and autophagy at the molecular level. These drugs are rapidly absorbed and accumulate primarily in granulocytes, erythrocytes, and thrombocytes. Notably, the concentration of CQ is up to seven times higher in the epidermis than in the dermis.

CQ and HCQ are known to have numerous immunomodulatory effects however, the exact mechanism is unknown. By altering lysosomal pH, antimalarials interfere with intracellular processing and diminish proteolysis and subsequent secretion of proteins within macrophages, dendritic cells and lymphocytes [62]. By altering lysosomal processing, antigen presentation via class II MHC is disrupted [63]. Leukocyte activation is diminished by antimalarial-induced inhibition of proinflammatory cytokines like TNF-α, IL-6, IL-1β, and IFN-γ [62, 64]. Furthermore, patients treated with CQ demonstrated increased numbers of lamellar inclusions in leukocytes which is associated with impaired chemotaxis, phagocytosis, and superoxide production by neutrophils [62, 65]. Antimalarials also demonstrate immunomodulation through endosomal inhibition of toll-like receptors (TLRs) [66]. Antimalarials have anti-inflammatory effects by inhibiting prostaglandin activity, leukotriene synthesis, and histamine release [67].

CQ and HCQ are used most commonly for autoimmune disorders in dermatology. Cutaneous disease in lupus erythematous (LE) responds well to HCQ including non-specific manifestations such as calcinosis cutis, ulceration, and panniculitis [68, 69]. This encompasses acute, subacute, and chronic cutaneous LE. HCQ therapy also improved systemic symptoms like fatigue and myalgia as well as decreased future flares of systemic disease [70, 71]. These effects are thought to be a result of few mechanisms including inhibition of lysosomal activation, decreased antigen presentation by major histocompatibility complex (MHC) Class II molecules, and chemotaxis inhibition. These mechanisms of antimalarial therapy can be applied similarly in the treatment of other autoimmune disorders such as dermatomyositis which results in improvement of cutaneous symptoms that are refractory to other systemic therapies [72].

Granulomatous disorders [73–75], lichen planus [76, 77], and chronic urticarial [78, 79] respond well to the anti-inflammatory effects of HCQ and CQ. This is primarily through a decrease of proinflammatory cytokines release, TLR inhibition, and decreased prostaglandin, histamine, and leukotriene activity [62]. Chronic urticaria is also improved through inhibition of antigen presentation by MHC Class II molecules [62, 80].

4.2 Levamisole

Levamisole acts as a nicotine acetylcholine receptor agonist that constantly stimulates helminths such as ascaris to induce muscular paralysis. It is readily absorbed and metabolized in the liver. Due to its severe side effect profile, levamisole was pulled from the United States market as a cancer drug in 2000. It is currently only approved in the United States for veterinary treatment.

Before its discontinuance, levamisole was used for its immunomodulatory effects in dermatologic disorders. Levamisole acts as an immunostimulatory. It restores T-cell function through cholinergic stimulation increasing lymphocyte cyclic guanosine monophosphate (cGMP) [81]. As a T cell adjuvant, levamisole upregulates T helper cells and associated interleukins including IL-2, IL-12, and IFN-γ [82]. It also enhances macrophage phagocytosis, boosts neutrophil adherence and chemotaxis, and increases antibody formation [83].

Levamisole has demonstrated increased immunostimulation beneficial for dermatologic conditions. It restores function in impaired T cells to mount an immune response in acne vulgaris [84]. In vitiligo, endogenous immunosuppressive factors are diminished, and B cell activity increases to decrease circulating immune complex levels [85]. In collagen vascular disease such as systemic LE, levamisole restores delayed hypersensitivity response and improves impaired T cell function [86, 87].

4.3 Ivermectin

Ivermectin is a synthetic macrolide endectocide intended to treat endoparasites and tropical parasitic disease. Ivermectin binds selectively to neurotransmitter receptors specific to the peripheral motor synapses of parasites. Pharmacokinetic studies demonstrate good bioavailability, and the side effect profile is relatively safe [88].

Recently, ivermectin has become a popular choice for treatment of rosacea. The effect is thought to be primarily through activity against *Demodex* mites. However, topical application of ivermectin has demonstrated anti-inflammatory effects through decreased neutrophil chemotaxis, inhibition of proinflammatory cytokines like IL-1α and TNF-α, and upregulation of anti-inflammatory IL-23. Clinical studies show greater clearance rates with use of topical ivermectin when compared to a placebo [89].

5 Conclusion

Antimicrobials are valuable tools for dermatologists when treating noninfectious dermatoses. Several antimicrobial drugs still have unclear mechanisms of action; however, the immunomodulatory and beneficial therapeutic effects are often well documented in clinical trials various pre-clinical models. Clinicians can leverage these drugs to effectively manage dermatologic conditions while minimizing side effects by using lower or pulsed dosages. Dermatologists, as leading prescribers of antibiotics, should be aware of the multifaceted effect these drugs can have and treat their patients accordingly.

References

1. Ritts RE. Antibiotics as biological response modifiers. J Antimicrob Chemotherap. 1990;26(suppl-C):31–36. https://doi.org/10.1093/jac/26.suppl_C.31
2. Pasquale TR, Tan JS. Nonantimicrobial effects of antibacterial agents. Clin Infect Dis. 2005;40(1):127–35. https://doi.org/10.1086/426545.
3. Outpatient Antibiotic Prescriptions—United States (2019).
4. Murphy CS, McKay G. Clindamycin. Pract Diabet. 2015;32(6):222–3a. https://doi.org/10.1002/pdi.1962
5. Barza M, Goldstein JA, Kane A, Feingold DS, Pochi PE. Systemic absorption of clindamycin hydrochloride after topical application. J Am Acad Dermatol. 1982;7(2):208–14. https://doi.org/10.1016/S0190-9622(82)70109-4.
6. van Hoogdalem EJ, Baven TLM, Spiegel-Melsen I, Terpstra IJ. Transdermal absorption of clindamycin and tretinoin from topically applied anti-acne formulations in man. Biopharm Drug Dispos. 1998;19(9):563–9. https://doi.org/10.1002/(SICI)1099-081X(199812)19:9%3c563::AID-BDD134%3e3.0.CO;2-E.
7. Whitney KM, Ditre CM. Anti-inflammatory properties of clindamycin: a review of its use in the treatment of acne vulgaris. Clinic Med Insights Dermatol. 2011;4:27. https://doi.org/10.4137/CMD.S5058.
8. van der Zee HH, Boer J, Prens EP, Jemec GBE. The effect of combined treatment with oral clindamycin and oral rifampicin in patients with hidradenitis suppurativa. Dermatology. 2009;219(2):143–7. https://doi.org/10.1159/000228337.
9. Cholo MC, Steel HC, Fourie PB, Germishuizen WA, Anderson R. Clofazimine: current status and future prospects. J Antimicrob Chemother. 2012;67(2):290–8. https://doi.org/10.1093/jac/dkr444.
10. Wozel G, Blasum C. Dapsone in dermatology and beyond. Arch Dermatol Res. 2014;306(2):103–24. https://doi.org/10.1007/s00403-013-1409-7.
11. Ghaoui N, Hanna E, Abbas O, Kibbi AG, Kurban M. Update on the use of dapsone in dermatology. Int J Dermatol. 2020;59(7):787–95. https://doi.org/10.1111/ijd.14761.
12. Wu L, Zhang W, Tian L, Bao K, Li P, Lin J. Immunomodulatory effects of erythromycin and its derivatives on human T-lymphocyte in vitro. Immunopharmacol Immunotoxicol. 2007;29(3–4):587–96. https://doi.org/10.1080/08923970701692841.

13. Labro MT. Anti-inflammatory activity of macrolides: a new therapeutic potential? J Antimicrob Chemother. 1998;41 Suppl B:37–46. https://doi.org/10.1093/jac/41.suppl_2.37
14. Polat M, Lenk N, Yalcin B, et al. Efficacy of erythromycin for psoriasis vulgaris. Clin Exp Dermatol. 2007;32(3):295–7. https://doi.org/10.1111/j.1365-2230.2007.02370.x.
15. Saxena VN, Dogra J. Long-term oral azithromycin in chronic plaque psoriasis: a controlled trial. Eur J Dermatol. 2010;20(3):329–33. https://doi.org/10.1684/ejd.2010.0930.
16. Sharma PK, Yadav TP, Gautam RK, Taneja N, Satyanarayana L. Erythromycin in pityriasis rosea: a double-blind, placebo-controlled clinical trial. J Am Acad Dermatol. 2000;42(2 Pt 1):241–4. https://doi.org/10.1016/S0190-9622(00)90132-4.
17. Pandhi D, Singal A, Verma P, Sharma R. The efficacy of azithromycin in pityriasis rosea: a randomized, double-blind, placebo-controlled trial. Indian J Dermatol Venereol Leprol. 2014;80(1):36–40. https://doi.org/10.4103/0378-6323.125484.
18. Truhan AP, Hebert AA, Esterly NB. Pityriasis lichenoides in children: therapeutic response to erythromycin. J Am Acad Dermatol. 1986;15(1):66–70. https://doi.org/10.1016/s0190-9622(86)70144-8.
19. Alzolibani AA, Zedan K. Macrolides in chronic inflammatory skin disorders. Mediators Inflamm. 2012;2012: 159354. https://doi.org/10.1155/2012/159354.
20. Edwards DI. Nitroimidazole drugs—action and resistance mechanisms. I. Mechanisms of action. J Antimicrob Chemother. 1993;31(1):9–20. https://doi.org/10.1093/jac/31.1.9
21. Lamp KC, Freeman CD, Klutman NE, Lacy MK. Pharmacokinetics and pharmacodynamics of the nitroimidazole antimicrobials. Clin Pharmacokinet. 1999;36(5):353–73. https://doi.org/10.2165/00003088-199936050-00004.
22. Akamatsu H, Oguchi M, Nishijima S, et al. The inhibition of free radical generation by human neutrophils through the synergistic effects of metronidazole with palmitoleic acid: a possible mechanism of action of metronidazole in rosacea and acne. Arch Dermatol Res. 1990;282(7):449–54. https://doi.org/10.1007/BF00402621.
23. Schmadel LK, McEvoy GK. Topical metronidazole: a new therapy for rosacea. Clin Pharm. 1990;9(2):94–101.
24. Parsad D, Pandhi R, Negi KS, Kumar B. Topical metronidazole in seborrheic dermatitis–a double-blind study. Dermatology. 2001;202(1):35–7. https://doi.org/10.1159/000051582.
25. Siadat AH, Iraji F, Shahmoradi Z, Enshaieh S, Taheri A. The efficacy of 1% metronidazole gel in facial seborrheic dermatitis: a double blind study. Indian J Dermatol Venereol Leprol. 2006;72(4):266–9. https://doi.org/10.4103/0378-6323.26745.
26. Spisani S, Traniello S, Martuccio C, Rizzuti O, Cellai L. Rifamycins inhibit human neutrophil functions: new derivatives with potential antiinflammatory activity. Inflammation. 1997;21(4):391–400. https://doi.org/10.1023/a:1027314419843.
27. Ziglam HM, Daniels I, Finch RG. Immunomodulating activity of rifampicin. J Chemother. 2004;16(4):357–61. https://doi.org/10.1179/joc.2004.16.4.357.
28. Dessinioti C, Zisimou C, Tzanetakou V, Stratigos A, Antoniou C. Oral clindamycin and rifampicin combination therapy for hidradenitis suppurativa: a prospective study and 1-year follow-up. Clin Exp Dermatol. 2016;41(8):852–7. https://doi.org/10.1111/ced.12933.
29. Tsankov N, Grozdev I, Kkzandjieva J. Old drug—new indication. Rifampicin in psoriasis. J Dermatol Treat. 2006;17(1):18–23. https://doi.org/10.1080/09546630500375643
30. Tsankov N, Grozdev I. Rifampicin—a mild immunosuppressive agent for psoriasis. J Dermatolog Treat. 2011;22(2):62–4. https://doi.org/10.3109/09546630903496975.
31. Mela M, Mancuso A, Burroughs AK. Review article: pruritus in cholestatic and other liver diseases. Aliment Pharmacol Ther. 2003;17(7):857–70. https://doi.org/10.1046/j.1365-2036.2003.01458.x.
32. Webster GMDP. Del Rosso JQDOF anti-inflammatory activity of tetracyclines. Dermatologic Clinic. 2007;25(2):133–5. https://doi.org/10.1016/j.det.2007.01.012.
33. Jantzie LLP, Todd KGP. Doxycycline inhibits proinflammatory cytokines but not acute cerebral cytogenesis after hypoxia–ischemia in neonatal rats. J Psychiatry Neurosci. 2010;35(1):20–32. https://doi.org/10.1503/jpn.090061.

34. Martin RR, Warr GA, Couch RB, Yeager H, Knight V. Effects of tetracycline on leukotaxis. J Infect Dis. 1974;129(2):110–6. https://doi.org/10.1093/infdis/129.2.110.
35. Perret LJ, Tait CP. Non-antibiotic properties of tetracyclines and their clinical application in dermatology. Australas J Dermatol. 2014;55(2):111–8. https://doi.org/10.1111/ajd.12075.
36. Golub LM, Ramamurthy NS, McNamara TF, Greenwald RA, Rifkin BR. Tetracyclines inhibit connective tissue breakdown: new therapeutic implications for an old family of drugs. Crit Rev Oral Biol Med. 1991;2(3):297–321. https://doi.org/10.1177/10454411910020030201.
37. Kraus RL, Pasieczny R, Lariosa-Willingham K, Turner MS, Jiang A, Trauger JW. Antioxidant properties of minocycline: neuroprotection in an oxidative stress assay and direct radical-scavenging activity. J Neurochem. 2005;94(3):819–27. https://doi.org/10.1111/j.1471-4159.2005.03219.x.
38. Webster GF, Toso SM, Hegemann L. Inhibition of a model of in vitro granuloma formation by tetracyclines and ciprofloxacin: involvement of protein kinase C. Arch Dermatol. 1994;130(6):748–52. https://doi.org/10.1001/archderm.1994.01690060078008.
39. Korting HC, Schöllmann C. Tetracycline actions relevant to rosacea treatment. Skin Pharmacol Physiol. 2009. https://doi.org/10.1159/000235550.
40. Del Rosso JQDO, Webster GFMDP, Jackson MMD, et al. Two randomized phase III clinical trials evaluating anti-inflammatory dose doxycycline (40-mg doxycycline, USP capsules) administered once daily for treatment of rosacea. J Am Acad Dermatol. 2007;56(5):791–802. https://doi.org/10.1016/j.jaad.2006.11.021
41. Toossi P, Farshchian M, Malekzad F, Mohtasham N, Kimyai-Asadi A. Subantimicrobial-dose doxycycline in the treatment of moderate facial acne. J Drugs Dermatol. 2008;7(12):1149–52.
42. The use of doxycycline in lichen planopilaris and frontal fibrosing alopecia: a retrospective study of 138 patients at a tertiary referral clinic. J Am Acad Dermatol. 2019;81(4):AB135. https://doi.org/10.1016/j.jaad.2019.06.509
43. Joshi RK, Atukorala DN, Abanmi A, Khamis O, Haleem A. Successful treatment of Sweet's syndrome with doxycycline. Br J Dermatol. 1993;128(5):584–6. https://doi.org/10.1111/j.1365-2133.1993.tb00242.x.
44. Koshy T, Binitha MP. Minocycline in Pyoderma gangrenosum. Indian J Dermatol Venereol Leprol. 1992;58(3):210–2.
45. Elewski BE. Mechanisms of action of systemic antifungal agents. J Am Acad Dermatol. 1993;28(5):S28–34. https://doi.org/10.1016/S0190-9622(09)80305-8.
46. Rosen T, Schell BJ, Orengo I. Anti-inflammatory activity of antifungal preparations. Int J Dermatol. 1997;36(10):788–92. https://doi.org/10.1046/j.1365-4362.1997.00309.x.
47. Gupta AK, Nicol K, Batra R. Role of antifungal agents in the treatment of seborrheic dermatitis. Am J Clin Dermatol. 2004;5(6):417–22. https://doi.org/10.2165/00128071-200405060-00006.
48. Elewski B, Ling MR, Phillips TJ. Efficacy and safety of a new once-daily topical ketoconazole 2% gel in the treatment of seborrheic dermatitis: a phase III trial. J Drugs Dermatol. 2006;5(7):646–50.
49. Borgers M, Degreef H, Vermeerbergen G. The role of ketoconazole in seborrheic dermatitis. Cutis. 2007;80(4):359–63.
50. Piérard GE, Piérard-Franchimont C, Van Cutsem J, Rurangirwa A, Hoppenbrouwers ML, Schrooten P. Ketoconazole 2% emulsion in the treatment of seborrheic dermatitis. Int J Dermatol. 1991;30(11):806–9. https://doi.org/10.1111/j.1365-4362.1991.tb04793.x.
51. Tsai Y-C, Tsai T-F. Itraconazole in the treatment of nonfungal cutaneous diseases: a review. Dermatol Therap. 2019;9(2):271–80. https://doi.org/10.1007/s13555-019-0299-9.
52. Mihara M, Hagari Y, Morimura T, et al. Itraconazole as a new treatment for pustulosis palmaris et plantaris. Arch Dermatol. 1998;134(5):639–40. https://doi.org/10.1001/archderm.134.5.639.
53. V'Lckova-Laskoska MT, Caca-Biljanovska NG, Laskoski DS, Kamberova SJ. Palmoplantar pustulosis treated with itraconazole: a single, active-arm pilot study. Dermatol Ther. 2009;22(1):85–9. https://doi.org/10.1111/j.1529-8019.2008.01219.x.
54. Khandpur S, Sugandhan S, Sharma VK. Pulsed itraconazole therapy in eruptive lichen planus. J Eur Acad Dermatol Venereol. 2009;23(1):98–101. https://doi.org/10.1111/j.1468-3083.2008.02743.x.

55. Pawelec G, Ehninger G, Rehbein A, Schaudt K, Jaschonek K. Comparison of the immunosuppressive activities of the antimycotic agents itraconazole, fluconazole, ketoconazole and miconazole on human T-cells. Int J Immunopharmacol. 1991;13(2):299–304. https://doi.org/10.1016/0192-0561(91)90111-J.
56. Cooper SM, Sheridan A, Burge S. Mycosis fungoides responding to systemic itraconazole. J Eur Acad Dermatol Venereol. 2003;17(5):588–90. https://doi.org/10.1046/j.1468-3083.2003.00763.x.
57. Kim J, Tang JY, Gong R, et al. Itraconazole, a commonly used antifungal that inhibits hedgehog pathway activity and cancer growth. Cancer Cell. 2010;17(4):388–99. https://doi.org/10.1016/j.ccr.2010.02.027.
58. Kim DJ, Kim J, Spaunhurst K, et al. Open-label, exploratory phase II trial of oral itraconazole for the treatment of basal cell carcinoma. J Clin Oncol. 2014;32(8):745–51. https://doi.org/10.1200/JCO.2013.49.9525.
59. Del Carratore R, Carpi A, Beffy P, et al. Itraconazole inhibits HMEC-1 angiogenesis. Biomed Pharmacother. 2011;66(4):312–7. https://doi.org/10.1016/j.biopha.2011.11.004.
60. Chapouly C, Guimbal S, Hollier P-L, Renault M-A. Role of hedgehog signaling in vasculature development, differentiation, and maintenance. Int J Mol Sci. 2019;20(12):3076. https://doi.org/10.3390/ijms20123076.
61. Bessar H, Kandil AH, Nasr NM, Khattab F. Itraconazole versus propranolol: therapeutic and pharmacologic effect on serum angiopoietin-2 in patients with infantile hemangioma. J Dermatolog Treat. 2022;33(1):105–10. https://doi.org/10.1080/09546634.2019.1687822.
62. Kalia S, Dutz JP. New concepts in antimalarial use and mode of action in dermatology. Dermatol Ther. 2007;20(4):160–74. https://doi.org/10.1111/j.1529-8019.2007.00131.x.
63. Nowell J, Quaranta V. Chloroquine affects biosynthesis of Ia molecules by inhibiting dissociation of invariant (gamma) chains from alpha-beta dimers in B cells. J Exp Med. 1985;162(4):1371–6. https://doi.org/10.1084/jem.162.4.1371.
64. van den Borne BE, Dijkmans BA, de Rooij HH, le Cessie S, Verweij CL. Chloroquine and hydroxychloroquine equally affect tumor necrosis factor-alpha, interleukin 6, and interferon-gamma production by peripheral blood mononuclear cells. J Rheumatol. 1997;24(1):55–60.
65. Hurst NP, French JK, Gorjatschko L, Betts WH. Chloroquine and hydroxychloroquine inhibit multiple sites in metabolic pathways leading to neutrophil superoxide release. J Rheumatol. 1988;15(1):23–7.
66. Kužnik A, Benčina M, Švajger U, Jeras M, Rozman B, Jerala R. Mechanism of endosomal TLR inhibition by antimalarial drugs and imidazoquinolines. J Immunol. 2011;186(8):4794–804. https://doi.org/10.4049/jimmunol.1000702.
67. Löffler BM, Bohn E, Hesse B, Kunze H. Effects of antimalarial drugs on phospholipase A and lysophospholipase activities in plasma membrane, mitochondrial, microsomal and cytosolic subcellular fractions of rat liver. Biochim Biophys Acta. 1985;835(3):448–55. https://doi.org/10.1016/0005-2760(85)90114-6.
68. Chasset F, Bouaziz JD, Costedoat-Chalumeau N, Francès C, Arnaud L. Efficacy and comparison of antimalarials in cutaneous lupus erythematosus subtypes: a systematic review and meta-analysis. Br J Dermatol. 2017;177(1):188–96. https://doi.org/10.1111/bjd.15312.
69. Tsakonas E, Joseph L, Esdaile JM, et al. A long-term study of hydroxychloroquine withdrawal on exacerbations in systemic lupus erythematosus Canadian Hydroxychloroquine Study Group. Lupus. 1998;7(2):80–5. https://doi.org/10.1191/096120398678919778.
70. Alarcón GS, McGwin G, Bertoli AM, et al. Effect of hydroxychloroquine on the survival of patients with systemic lupus erythematosus: data from LUMINA, a multiethnic US cohort (LUMINA L). Ann Rheum Dis. 2007;66(9):1168–72. https://doi.org/10.1136/ard.2006.068676.
71. Fessler BJ, Alarcón GS, McGwin G, et al. Systemic lupus erythematosus in three ethnic groups: XVI. Association of hydroxychloroquine use with reduced risk of damage accrual. Arthritis Rheum. 2005;52(5):1473–80. https://doi.org/10.1002/art.21039
72. Woo TY, Callen JP, Voorhees JJ, Bickers DR, Hanno R, Hawkins C. Cutaneous lesions of dermatomyositis are improved by hydroxychloroquine. J Am Acad Dermatol. 1984;10(4):592–600. https://doi.org/10.1016/s0190-9622(84)80263-7.

73. Cannistraci C, Lesnoni La Parola I, Falchi M, Picardo M. Treatment of generalized granuloma annulare with hydroxychloroquine. Dermatology. 2005;211(2):167–8. https://doi.org/10.1159/000086452
74. Simon M, von den Driesch P. Antimalarials for control of disseminated granuloma annulare in children. J Am Acad Dermatol. 1994;31(6):1064–5. https://doi.org/10.1016/s0190-9622(09)80089-3.
75. Jones E, Callen JP. Hydroxychloroquine is effective therapy for control of cutaneous sarcoidal granulomas. J Am Acad Dermatol. 1990;23(3 Pt 1):487–9. https://doi.org/10.1016/0190-9622(90)70246-e.
76. Eisen D. Hydroxychloroquine sulfate (Plaquenil) improves oral lichen planus: an open trial. J Am Acad Dermatol. 1993;28(4):609–12. https://doi.org/10.1016/0190-9622(93)70082-5.
77. Raj SC, Baral D, Garhnayak L, et al. Hydroxychloroquine-a new treatment option for erosive oral lichen planus. Indian J Dent Res. 2021;32(2):192–8. https://doi.org/10.4103/ijdr.IJDR_943_20.
78. Boonpiyathad T, Sangasapaviliya A. Hydroxychloroquine in the treatment of anti-histamine refractory chronic spontaneous urticaria, randomized single-blinded placebo-controlled trial and an open label comparison study. Eur Ann Allergy Clin Immunol. 2017;49(5):220–4. https://doi.org/10.23822/EurAnnACI.1764-1489.11.
79. Reeves GE, Boyle MJ, Bonfield J, Dobson P, Loewenthal M. Impact of hydroxychloroquine therapy on chronic urticaria: chronic autoimmune urticaria study and evaluation. Intern Med J. 2004;34(4):182–6. https://doi.org/10.1111/j.1444-0903.2004.00532.x.
80. Haas N, Iwen W, Grabbe J, Uchanska-Ziegler B, Czarnetzki BM. MHC class II antigen expression is increased in different forms of urticaria. Int Arch Allergy Immunol. 1996;109(2):177–82. https://doi.org/10.1159/000237217.
81. Scheinfeld N, Rosenberg JD, Weinberg JM. Levamisole in dermatology: a review. Am J Clin Dermatol. 2004;5(2):97–104. https://doi.org/10.2165/00128071-200405020-00004.
82. Szeto C, Gillespie KM, Mathieson PW. Levamisole induces interleukin-18 and shifts type 1/type 2 cytokine balance. Immunology. 2000;100(2):217–24. https://doi.org/10.1046/j.1365-2567.2000.00042.x.
83. Renoux G. The general immunopharmacology of levamisole. Drugs. 1980;20(2):89–99. https://doi.org/10.2165/00003495-198020020-00001.
84. De Cree J, De Cock W, Verhaegen H. Levamisole treatment of inflammatory acne: restoration of impaired T-cell function accompanied by clearing of the lesions. Biomedicine. 1979;31(4):95–9.
85. Khondker L, Khan SI. Efficacy of levamisole for the treatment of slow spreading vitiligo. Mymensingh Med J. 2013;22(4):761–6.
86. Gandzha IM, Sakharchuk VM, Lysenko GI, Mironova KA, Galetskaia TM. Use of levamisole in the adjuvant therapy of rheumatoid arthritis and systemic lupus erythematosus. Vrach Delo. 1981;2:16–8.
87. Rovenský J, Zitňan D, Cebecauer L, Lukác J. Our experiences with levamisole treatment in systemic lupus erythematosus (author's transl). Bratisl Lek Listy. 1981;75(5):603–10.
88. Dourmishev AL, Dourmishev LA, Schwartz RA. Ivermectin: pharmacology and application in dermatology. Int J Dermatol. 2005;44(12):981–8. https://doi.org/10.1111/j.1365-4632.2004.02253.x.
89. Cardwell LA, Alinia H, MoradiTuchayi S, Feldman SR. New developments in the treatment of rosacea—role of once-daily ivermectin cream. Clin Cosmet Investig Dermatol. 2016;9:71–7. https://doi.org/10.2147/CCID.S98091.

Integrative Therapies as Immunomodulators

Nicole Naterelli, Nimrit Gahoonia, and Raja K. Sivamani

Abstract The field of integrative medicine is rapidly advancing and, given the multidisciplinary approach as well as influences from many parts of the world, brings together many facets of immunology and immunomodulation. The diverse origins of therapies, including herbal, botanical, spice roots, and other natural sources, give rise to many applications as anti-inflammatory agents. Dermatologists incorporate integrative therapies in diseases such as acne, rosacea, atopic dermatitis, psoriasis, and hidradenitis suppurativa among others, attempting to modulate the actions of neurotransmitters, cytokines, and cellular balances. More importantly, the advances in the field are highlighting combination therapies as well as alternatives to prescription medicines to accomplish therapeutic benefits. This chapter will outline the impact of diet and nutrition, supplementation, and probiotics, used in conjunction with or without conventional immunomodulators to modify a disease process and bring benefits to patients who might have been previously out of options.

Keywords Probiotic · Gut · Botanical · Supplement · Holistic · Integrative · Inflammatory · Microbiome

---

N. Naterelli
Morsani College of Medicine, University of South Florida, 560 Channelside Drive, Tampa, FL 33602, USA

N. Gahoonia
Touro University College of Osteopathic Medicine, 1310 Club Dr, Vallejo, CA 94592, USA

R. K. Sivamani (✉)
College of Medicine, California Northstate University, 9700 W Taron Dr, Elk Grove, CA 95757, USA
e-mail: raja.sivamani.md@gmail.com

Integrative Skin Science and Research, 1495 River Park Drive, Sacramento, CA 95819, USA

Pacific Skin Institute, 1495 River Park Dr Suite 200, Sacramento, CA 95815, USA

Department of Dermatology, University of California-Davis, 3301 C St #1400, Sacramento, CA 95816, USA

N. Bhatia (ed.), *Immunomodulators and Biologics in Dermatologic Treatment*,
https://doi.org/10.1007/978-3-031-66590-5_9

Abbreviations

APC	Antigen presenting cell
cAMP	Cyclic adenosine monophosphate
FDA	Food and drug administration
HS	Hidradenitis suppurativa
ICI	Immune checkpoint inhibitor
JAK	Janus kinase
PDE-4	Phosphodiesterase-4
STAT	Signal transducer and activator
TNF	Tumor necrosis factor

1 Herbs, Probiotics, Nutrition and Inflammatory Disease

Although JAK inhibitors, biologics, and PDE-4 inhibitors have proven pivotal in treating many chronic inflammatory diseases within dermatology, they are associated with long-term use or side effects which may lead a patient to discontinue their use. Thus, this feature highlights the importance of targeting treatment approaches in a diverse way. As a result, much research has been performed towards identifying the most optimal types of diets, supplements, and herbal remedies unique to alleviating each inflammatory disease due to their immunomodulatory effects and will be the topic of discussion in this chapter.

1.1 Acne

Acne vulgaris is an inflammatory disorder of hair follicles and sebaceous glands, characterized by closed or open comedones, pustules, papules, and/or deep nodules [1]. An estimated 85% of individuals are affected within their lifetime [2], making acne the most common dermatologic condition diagnosed in the United States [1]. First line treatments for acne vulgaris include benzoyl peroxide, topical or oral retinoids, and topical or oral antibiotics. However, such management strategies are associated with a plethora of potential side effects, such as erythema, dryness, itching, stinging, and scaling [3, 4]. In addition, oral approaches can have systemic effects, such as epistaxis, hyperlipidemia, joint pain, teratogenicity with oral retinoids [5], and nausea, vomiting, diarrhea, hypersensitivity reactions with oral antibiotics [6], in addition to alteration of the gastrointestinal microflora.

1.1.1 Probiotics and Acne

As conventional treatments for acne vulgaris are associated with potential side effects, there is great interest in integrative approaches for the management of acne, such as dietary strategies and pre- or probiotics. Probiotics are living, commensal microorganisms that provide health benefits when consumed orally or applied topically. Probiotics have been implicated for the management of acne, as acne is associated with increased colonization of the bacteria *Cutibacterium acnes* [7]. In addition to introducing beneficial microorganisms into the gut or skin, probiotics, such as strains of *Lactobacilli,* have been shown to directly inhibit the growth of *C. acnes* in vitro [8]. In addition, a growing body of evidence further suggests that probiotics have immunomodulatory actions via the activation of T cells and the release of cytokines [9].

Oral Probiotics for Acne

Oral probiotics have been demonstrated to exhibit systemic anti-inflammatory effects [10]. For example, Lactobacillus strains have been shown to inhibit the proliferative activity of CD-4 + T cells, induce anti-inflammatory cytokines IL-10 and TGF-beta, and promote T-regulatory cell function [11]. In addition, strains such as *Streptococcus salivarius* and *Lactococcus* have been shown to directly inhibit the growth of *P. acnes* via the production of bacteriocins or bacteriocin-like inhibitory substances [12, 13].

Researchers have demonstrated interest in the effects of oral probiotics on acne vulgaris since the 1960s, when physician Robert H. Silver conducted the first clinical trial with 300 patients, albeit limited by lack of placebo controls [10]. Similarly, in 1987, Italian researchers conducted a study in which 20 patients received standard treatment, whereas 20 patients additionally received a probiotic adjuvant consisting of *Lactobacillus acidophilus* and *Bifidobacterium bifidum* [14]. Those receiving adjuvant probiotic treatment demonstrated better clinical outcomes and resolution of lesions in comparison to the group receiving standard treatment.

In addition, a 2013 study observed significant improvements in non-inflamed acne lesion counts every four weeks for twelve treatment weeks among patients receiving probiotics alone, minocycline alone, and combination treatment [15]. However, the authors found probiotic supplementation in combination with minocycline to significantly decrease total lesion count compared to groups receiving only probiotics ($p < 0.001$) or only minocycline ($0 < 0.01$). This suggests that oral probiotic supplementation may work effectively as a dual therapy, in combination with antibiotics.

Topical Probiotics for Acne

Recently, attention has been turned to the exploration of topical probiotics for the management of acne vulgaris. Topical probiotics have been demonstrated to impact skin barrier function and elicit antimicrobial properties [10]. A 2018 pilot study assessed the efficacy of a topical probiotic containing equal parts *L. rhamnosus* GG, *L. plantarum* WCFS1 and *L. pentosus* KCA1 on clinical improvement of acne [16]. Facial application twice daily for eight weeks resulted in reduction of inflammatory lesions and comedone formation compared to controls. Interestingly, the cutaneous microbiome composition temporarily shifted, resulting in a reduced relative abundance of *staphylococci* and *C. acnes*, and an increased relative abundance of *lactobacilli*.

A 2009 clinical trial observed a reduction of inflammatory lesions following application of *Enterococcus fecalis* lotion daily for 8 weeks [17]. Compared to the control group receiving a placebo lotion, those receiving the topical probiotic lotion exhibited a 50% reduction of inflammatory lesions. A 2012 clinical trial observed a reduction in acne lesion size and erythema with application of topical 5% *Lactobacillus plantarum* extract [18]. However, as efficacious results were not replicated with 1% extract, the beneficial effects of antimicrobial peptide-producing topical probiotics may be dose dependent.

1.1.2 Exacerbating and Alleviating Foods in Acne

Dairy

Dairy has long been theorized to be a culprit in the exacerbation of acne. Research has shown that consumption of milk can increase levels of insulin-like-growth factor-1 (IGF-1) [19]. In regards to acne specifically, IGF-1 causes increases in cutaneous androgen production and proliferation of sebaceous gland follicles which each contribute to the pathogenesis of acne [19, 20]. Thus, to understand the effects of this clinically, many large observational studies have been conducted to understand the strength of this relationship.

A cross sectional study performed via an online self-questionnaire with 24,452 participants aimed to understand acne and diet [21]. A significant relationship was found between active acne and consumption of milk (adjusted odds ratio 1.12). Another retrospective study evaluated 47,355 women with teenage acne and their consumption of milk [22]. The results displayed prevalence ratios of 1.12, 1.16, 1.44 for whole milk, low fat milk, and skim milk, respectively. The association to acne was strongest with skim milk suggesting that the addition of whey protein in most skim milks may be especially aggravating for acne [22]. Many additional observational studies have presented similar findings suggesting a strong relationship between acne and milk consumption [20]. Although no randomized double blind placebo controlled trials have been conducted to establish causation, it can still be reasonably concluded that a diet that excludes milk may be therapeutic for acne [20].

Chocolate

The belief that chocolate consumption exacerbates acne is widely controversial. This can be attributed to the reason that very few clinical trials have even explored the relationship between acne and chocolate, despite the popular assumption that chocolate aggravates acne [23]. Of these few trials, their findings cannot be fully generalizable due to their small sample sizes [24, 25] and short intervention durations [24, 26].

For instance, a randomized, double blind study conducted in 2014 with 14 males assessed the consumption of a one time binge consumption of 6 oz unsweetened 100-percent cocoa, 6 oz hydrolyzed gelatin powder, or a combination of both with varying cocoa dose (1, 2, 3, 4, or 5 oz) and the remaining hydrolyzed gelatin dose adjusted accordingly to achieve a total combination dose of 6 oz [24]. The study showed that acne lesions did significantly increase by day 7 ($p = 0.047$), however, the results did not indicate the differences in lesion counts across the various dosages of cacao given. Additionally, the sample size was too small and the study excluded women making the findings from this study not reliable to generalize to all patients with acne.

More recently, a study conducted in 2016 aimed to address the many flaws of previously conducted trials to present a more clear understanding. The trial was designed to be a single blind, randomized crossover study in which 54 students were recruited [27]. Participants were randomly assigned to consume 15 Jelly Belly jellybeans or a 45 g Hershey's milk chocolate bar (both provided the same glycemic load). Acne lesions were assessed at baseline and 48 h after consumption. Significant increases in acne lesions were noted in the chocolate consumption group compared to the jellybean group ($p < 0.0001$). They also found that this was also true across all genders, ages, and initial severity of acne. Additionally they showed that covariates such as age, stress, and gender had no statistically significant effects on the number of lesions. Thus, despite this study improving some aspects of the previously described studies, it is still difficult to conclude any well supported clinical guidance from the study. Therefore, among the very few research trials that have investigated the effects of chocolate on acne, it is still very unclear whether a direct relationship between chocolate consumption and worsening acne exists.

Low Glycemic Diet

The glycemic index is a scale which indicated the level of postprandial glucose concentrations after consumption of foods containing carbohydrates [28]. Low glycemic foods are considered those with a glycemic index below 55 [28]. These include foods such as fruits, vegetables, legumes, and nuts [29]. Research has shown that adhering to a diet consisting of low glycemic index foods may improve acne.

To assess the low glycemic diet a randomized controlled trial conducted a study with 43 male participants with mild to moderate acne for 12 weeks [30]. They instructed the participants to either consume a low glycemic diet (LGD) or carbohydrate rich foods with no reference to glycemic index. The LGD group was specifically defined as receiving "25% of energy from protein, 45% from low GI carbohydrates, and 30% energy from fats." At the end of the study, results showed a statistically significant decrease in total acne lesion counts in the LGD group ($p = 0.03$) and greater decreases in weight than the control group ($p < 0.001$).

Another randomized trial conducted in 2012 also evaluated the impacts of a low glycemic index diet [31]. Participants in the low glycemic index group were instructed to adhere to the same diet outlined previously by Smith et al. Examples of low glycemic index foods given were barley, whole grain breads, fish, fruits, and vegetables. The control group was instructed to consume carbohydrate rich foods. After 10 weeks, the treatment group had significant average decreases in acne lesion counts from baseline ($p = 0.02$). Compared to the control group, the decrease in lesion counts in the treatment group was also significant ($p = 0.02$).

Overall, consuming a low glycemic diet may be beneficial for those suffering from mild to moderate acne. The relationship of the diet to acne still needs further evaluation as it is unclear if there is any therapeutic benefit for those with more severe acne. Nevertheless, these small studies display promising results and may be a useful approach to augmenting first line acne therapies.

2 Psoriasis

Psoriasis is a chronic inflammatory dermatologic condition that affects almost 3% of the US adult population [32]. Many variants of psoriasis exist, however the predominant form is plaque psoriasis. Plaque psoriasis presents with thickened and well-demarcated erythematous plaques with silvery scaling that can be itchy [33]. Often these plaques develop on the extensor surfaces of the skin, scalp, trunk and limbs [33]. Multiple comorbidities exist with the development of psoriasis including: psoriatic arthritis, inflammatory bowel disease, cardiovascular disease, and mood disorders [34]. As a result, psoriasis has a profound burden and impact on the quality of life in patients with psoriasis.

The pathophysiology, although not fully understood, is believed to be attributed to a dysregulation of the immune system which ultimately leads to hyperproliferation of keratinocytes. Hyperproliferation results from a stressor that causes keratinocytes to release self-nucleotides and antimicrobial peptides [35]. This then recruits dendritic cells to release IL-23. IL-23 further upregulates Th17 cells which subsequently cause secretion of additional inflammatory cytokines including IL-17, IL-21, IL-23 and TNF-alpha [35]. Of particular importance, IL-17, has been noted to directly activate additional keratinocytes which will further magnify the inflammatory cascade by releasing additional inflammatory substances [35, 36]. This recurrent activation pattern of keratinocytes leads to the maintenance of the chronic pathology in psoriasis. Thus, many treatment options have targeted specific steps in the pathogenesis to prevent inflammation. These include use of ultraviolet (UV) irradiation, corticosteroids, IL-17 and IL-23 inhibitors and TNF-alpha inhibitors [37].

Due to the profound impacts and comorbidities that psoriasis can present with, it is important to take a multi-dimensional approach to hinder the feed-forward inflammatory pathway. Nutrition can play a vital role in this pathway. Several foods have been documented to have anti-inflammatory properties making diet an important factor to consider in psoriasis. Although diet is not a sole cure for psoriasis, it has proven to augment first line treatments [38].

2.1 Low Calorie Diet and Weight Loss

The effects of a low calorie diet (LCD) has been popularly researched in patients with psoriasis. One study conducted on patients with psoriasis and obesity found that a diet restricted to 800–1000 kcal/day for 8 weeks followed by an 8 week reintroduction to a normal diet of 1200 kcal/day resulted in a significant reduction in the Psoriasis Area and Severity Index (PASI) by $-$ 2.0 ($p = 0.06$) and an average weight loss of 16.4 kg ($p < 0.001$) compared to the control group at 16 weeks [39]. A similar study also showed that a LCD of less than 1000 kcal/day for 8 weeks led to PASI 75 by 85.9% in the diet group ($p < 0.001$) and an average weight loss of 12.9 kg [40]. Another study also displayed PASI 75 in 66.7% of the diet group after 24 week implementation of a LCD ($p < 0.001$) [41]. All three of these studies were conducted in patients with psoriasis and obesity suggesting that implementing a LCD that results in weight loss could greatly improve the severity of psoriasis, especially in patient that are overweight.

Independently, obesity is a chronic disease that causes low grade systemic inflammation. Adipose tissue is known to release many pro-inflammatory cytokines including TNF-alpha, IL-6, IL-12, IL-23 and causes activation of Th1 and Th17 cells, collectively increasing inflammation in the body [42]. When coupled with the inflammatory pathway occurring in psoriasis, it can be especially catastrophic on the body [39]. Thus, the management of obesity through weight loss can be said to dampen part of the ongoing inflammation in patients with psoriasis as demonstrated through the improvements in PASI seen in the aforementioned studies.

2.2 Dietary Supplements for Psoriasis

The impact of common fish oil supplements has been explored in patients with psoriasis. Fish oil supplements contain eicosapentaenoic acid (EPA), docosahexaenoic acid (DHA), and alpha-linolenic acid (ALA) which are all considered types of omega-3 polyunsaturated fats and have been associated with anti-inflammatory effects. Thus, assessing the effects on psoriasis has become of interest. A study conducted on 83 patients with chronic plaque psoriasis with a minimum score of 15 on PASI were randomly assigned to receive omega 3 daily infusions or omega 6 daily infusions for 2 weeks. Results showed that those receiving omega 3 infusion had a decreased PASI score by 11.2 ± 9.8 and the omega 6 group had a 7.5 ± 8.8 PASI decrease ($p = 0.048$) [43]. Another study also showed decreased average PASI scores compared to baseline at 4 weeks and 8 weeks of 1122 mg/day of EPA ethyl ester and 756 mg/day of DCA ethyl ester administration [44]. Despite some trials displaying therapeutic effects of fish oil on psoriasis, some studies have also shown no effect. For instance, one study conducted on 25 patients with plaque psoriasis found no significant difference in the severity of the psoriasis between fish oil supplementation vs olive oil supplementation [45]. Thus, although there may be some beneficial effect of fish oil supplementation on psoriasis, further investigation is warranted in larger sample sizes to develop a more clear understanding.

The implications of various other dietary supplements such as vitamin D, selenium, zinc and tryptophan have also been explored, however the therapeutic effects of each of these has been unclear due to the lack of consistent findings after supplementation [38]. As a result, increased research in the individual dietary supplementation of vitamins, minerals, or amino acids is required before any recommendations can be confidently made.

2.3 Topical Botanical Agents

A variety of botanical topical agents have been researched for their immunomodulatory effects on psoriasis lesions. According to a 2017 systematic review, the main botanicals investigated include *Mahonia aquifolium*, indigo naturalis, and aloe vera [46].

Six trials were summarized each showing significant improvements in psoriatic lesions with *Mahonia aquifolium* cream application. Some trials compared the efficacy of *Mahonia aquifolium* cream to prescription topical medications such as calcipotriol, tazarotene, and fluticasone propionate; results showed equal and in some cases, superior, efficacy in treating psoriatic lesions [46]. Interestingly, a trial conducted by Augustin et al. found that *Mahonia aquifolium* cream displayed epidermal and dermal decreases in T-cell infiltration highlighting its immunomodulatory effects on psoriasis [47].

The review summarized three trials conducted by Lin et al. and each displayed significant improvements of psoriasis lesions and one trial also showed 74% of patients in the indigo naturalis treatment group reached PASI 75. Additionally, there were no significant differences in the effects between crude or refined indigo naturalis ointment [46, 48]. Indigo naturalis was also found to significantly reduce NAPSI scores suggesting it has therapeutic effects on nail manifestations as well.

Aloe vera was also found to be consistently very beneficial among the six trials reviewed [46]. For instance, in a study conducted by Syed et al., participants in the 0.5% aloe vera treatment group experienced 76% improvements in their baseline

PASI score [49]. Most of these trials however were conducted in patients who had mild to moderate plaque psoriasis, so more research is required to determine if aloe vera would be as beneficial in those with a higher severity.

In general, many botanical therapies have been proven to be efficacious in the treatment of psoriasis. Although more research is required to determine the extent of their benefits in the various types of psoriasis, it is promising to note that they are effective in mild to moderate plaque psoriasis. Thus, this presents another useful treatment modality clinicians can use to boost effects of more standard treatments.

2.4 Hidradenitis Suppurativa (HS)

Hidradenitis Suppurativa (HS) is a debilitating autoinflammatory skin disease that can greatly impact one's quality of life. HS is characterized by large and painful pimple-like bumps due to cellular overgrowth, which clogs hair follicles and sweat glands and results in inflammation. The precise cause of HS remains unknown, although experts believe there may be a variety of contributing factors, such as hormones, genetic disposition, cigarette smoking, and excess weight. There is no cure for HS, although treatment is necessary for symptom management and the prevention of permanent scarring. Conventional treatments may include topical or oral antibiotics, intralesional corticosteroids, or biologics [50].

2.4.1 Brewer's Yeast Exclusion Diet

Brewer's yeast (BY) is a common additive that is used in the production of beer and bakery items. BY is composed of a single celled fungus called *Saccharomyces cerevisiae*. Interestingly, anti-*Saccharomyces cerevisiae* antibodies have been found in patients with inflammatory diseases such as Crohn's disease, spondyloarthritis, and HS [51]. Thus, this finding presented a unique opportunity to target treatment approaches for HS.

A prospective study following 12 patients were instructed to follow a brewer's yeast exclusion diet for 1 year after receiving standard treatments as recommended based on their HS severity (surgical excision, debridement, etc.). Patients were instructed to exclude all bakery products, vinegar, black tea, soy sauces, beer, wine, cereals containing yeast and fermented cheese from their diet [52]. The recommended diet was consuming fresh fruits and vegetables, white meats, eggs, green tea, and coffee [52]. Results showed that all clinical symptoms had resolved with complete regression of previous skin lesions. Self reports from patients indicated that any accidental consumption of brewer's yeast caused immediate return of skin lesions [52]. All patients in the study were found to have IgG reactions to anti-*Saccharomyces cerevisiae* antigens. Therefore, the success of a brewer's yeast exclusion diet can be explained by the decreased likelihood of antigen-antibody complex formation thereby evading heightened levels of inflammation in HS.

An additional study in 2020 further solidified this correlation. The researchers asked 37 patients to follow the same diet as outlined in the previous study and were followed over a period of 6 years [53]. Overall, 70% of the patients reported, via a questionnaire, an improvement in their HS symptoms without any other treatments. Additionally 87% reported exacerbations of their symptoms after eating an excluded food within a few days of consumption [53].

Overall, making modifications in diet for those suffering with HS is an essential component for any effective treatment plan. Although dietary modifications do not exclusively constitute a cure for HS, it is an undeniably synergistic component to augment traditional treatments.

2.4.2 Supplements and Vitamins

In addition to conventional treatment, researchers have assessed the efficacy of nutritional supplements including riboflavin, vitamin D, and zinc gluconate on the clinical improvement of HS [54]. A 1960 case-series evaluated oral supplementation with riboflavin three times daily on the disappearance of HS-associated lesions [55]. The authors observed disappearance of lesions in all cases at 3 year follow-up and noted that supplementation could be stopped without relapse. Brocard et al. (2007) assessed the efficacy of zinc gluconate oral supplementation among 22 HS patients who were refractory to prior treatment [56]. In addition, 36% of subjects experienced complete remission. However, upon dose reduction from 90 mg daily to 30–60 mg daily, relapse occurred, although reversed upon dose increase. All of the remaining subjects experienced partial remission. Another study conducted on patients with mild to moderate HS studied the effects of oral zinc and nicotinamide supplements as a maintenance therapy after treating patients with oral minocycline 100 mg daily for 12 weeks previously. Those in the treatment group consumed the supplements daily for 90 days and the control group received no supplementation. Significant reductions in the International HS Severity Score System were found at 12 and 24 weeks in the treatment group compared to control ($p < 0.005$) [57].

A 2015 study assessed the effects of vitamin D supplementation among 14 HS patients who had undergone no prior treatment [58]. Vitamin D was individually dosed based on deficiency, and the number of nodules and flare-ups were assessed. At month 6, the authors observed a significant reduction in nodule number ($p = 0.01133$). In addition, 79% of patients achieved therapeutic success, defined as a reduction in the number of nodules and the frequency of flare-ups by at least 20%. Collectively, these results depict the potential utility of nutritional supplements and vitamins for the management of HS. However, all three reports are limited by the omission of a control group and small sample sizes.

2.4.3 Probiotics

Although the pathogenic model of HS is shifting to an autoinflammatory keratinization disease regulated by important cytokines [59], recent research has suggested the potential role of the microbiome. A 2020 study assessed the cutaneous microbiome among 30 HS patients and 24 healthy control subjects via next-generation sequencing targeting 16S and 18S ribosomal DNA. 48 HS lesional skin microbiomes consisted predominantly of *Corynebacterium, Porphyromonas,* and *Peptoniphilus* species, with an absence of *Cutibacterium acnes.* In contrast, *Porphyromonas,* and *Peptoniphilus* species were not detected in control samples. Interestingly, the authors compared lesional vs. nonlesional skin of HS patients and noted a significantly reduced relative abundance of *Propionibacterium* species and *C. acnes* in lesional skin, leading the authors to hypothesize that a reduction of *Propionibacterium* may contribute to the pathogenesis of HS. Although *C. acnes* contributes to the pathogenesis of acne vulgaris, the resulting dysbiosis in HS lesion skin may be associated with strophic sebaceous glands with reduced sebum excretion rate, characteristic of HS [60].

In general, studies assessing the microbiome of HS patients consistently suggest an increased relative abundance of anaerobic gram negative bacteria including *Porphyromonas,* and *Prevotella* species. Via the upregulation of antimicrobial peptides, these microbiota are postulated to catalyze inflammatory cascades and increase keratinocyte proliferation [60, 61]. Microbiome dysbiosis and characteristic microbiota signatures have led researchers to consider the utility of probiotics for the management of HS. [62] suggest topical probiotics may restore microbial composition via the replenishment of *Corynebacterium* spp., *Staphylococcus epidermidis,* and *Cutibacterium acnes* [84]. However, future clinical studies are required to validate current hypotheses regarding the potential role of topical and oral probiotics.

2.5 *Rosacea*

Rosacea is a chronic inflammatory disease characterized by facial erythema, flushing, and telangiectasia, with some subtypes additionally presenting with papules, pustules, and fibrosis [63]. Rosacea is a common skin disease, affecting about 5% of the adult population globally [64]. However, prevalence is greatest among those with lighter skin and advancing age [63]. Although there is no cure, therapeutic strategies can reduce symptoms, improve quality of life and prevent progression [65].

FDA approved topical treatments include metronidazole 0.75% and 1% gel or cream, encapsulated benzoyl peroxide 5% cream, azelaic acid 15% gel, and ivermectin 1% cream. In addition, the FDA has approved brimonidine tartrate 0.33% gel and oxymetazoline 1% cream, which are selective α2-adrenergic receptor agonists but with no inflammatory actions [71]. Systemic antibiotic therapy may be warranted for individuals with severe rosacea, although with risk of side effects from prolonged use, such as the growth of resistant microorganisms [69]. Laser and light therapies indicated for erythema and telangiectasia are limited by their associated cost.

2.5.1 Topical Botanicals

Botanical therapies and other natural products are becoming increasingly popular for a variety of skin diseases. Botanical and herbal remedies may be more cost effective, with reduced incidence of antibiotic-associated adverse effects. However, transient burning, pruritus, and even hypersensitivity reactions are possible [63].

A 2005 randomized controlled trial assessed the efficacy of *Chrysanthellum indicum* 1% extract cream compared to vehicle control among 246 subjects [66]. *Chrysanthellum indicum* is a plant extract that contains phenylpropanoic acids, flavonoids, and saponosides, with reported effects on vascular permeability and resistance. Although the authors noted no significant difference in the area of rosacea involvement between treatment groups, those receiving the extract cream depicted significant improvement in erythema and severity compared to the placebo group.

Quassia amara 4% extract gel has also been assessed for the reduction of papule or pustule count, flushing severity, and telangiectasia severity associated with rosacea [67]. Significant reductions of all three outcome measures were observed compared to baseline. Interestingly, those with severe rosacea depicted the greatest improvement.

Studies have also assessed the effects of botanical adjuvants in combination with standard therapy. While Broniarczyk-Dyla et al. (2011) observed a significant reduction in erythema severity and transepidermal water loss with licochalcone cream monotherapy [68], a prior study assessed the efficacy of licochalcone cream in conjunction with metronidazole [69]. They observed a significant improvement of erythema, in addition to symptoms including burning, stinging, itching, and tingling after two and four weeks, compared to baseline. However, both studies are limited by their omission of a control group.

However, a 2006 randomized controlled trial observed efficacious results following 8-week treatment with an herbal chibixiao recipe in combination with minocycline and spironolactone [70]. The control group only received antibiotic treatment. Clinical erythema, capillary dilation, and papule and pustule count was significantly reduced in the group receiving combination treatment compared to the control group. However, it is necessary to note that cryotherapy was additionally used in both groups.

A 2015 systematic review evaluated phytochemical and botanical therapies for rosacea, including the previously discussed studies with six additional published manuscripts and two poster abstracts [63]. Ultimately, they found botanicals to be the most effective in the improvement of facial erythema and papule and pustule counts. *Quassia amara* extract was the only botanical efficacious in the improvement of telangiectasia. In contrast, other botanicals such as silymarin and niacinamide cream were ineffective in improving the appearance of telangiectasias [63]. Ultimately, however, these studies depict the promising use of botanicals for the management of rosacea, especially among those who may be sensitive or refractory to conventional therapy.

2.6 *Atopic Dermatitis*

Atopic dermatitis (AD) is a chronic inflammatory dermatologic disorder that presents most commonly during infancy, although adult onset can occur as well. AD typically causes patients to experience pruritus that leads to significant redness, dryness, and irritation [71]. Often the rash can present on the scalp, face and other flexor surfaces of the skin. Depending on the severity, the quality of life in patients suffering from AD can be greatly diminished as the rashes can often be extremely persistent and remitting. The pathophysiology of AD is complex and with many contributing factors including: dysregulated immune responses, altered skin barrier, and IgE mediated hypersensitivity [72]. Current first line treatment is topical corticosteroids [73]. Additional alternative treatments include topical PDE4 inhibitors, ultraviolet phototherapy, topical calcineurin inhibitors and moisturizing creams [73]. Although there are multiple treatment options, none constitute a cure and flare ups are common in AD. Thus, finding additional therapies to improve symptoms and quality of life have been investigated.

2.6.1 Probiotics

The use of probiotics has been well investigated in AD. Although there has been no one consensus among the findings of each study, the use of probiotics may still be beneficial for some individuals. The most commonly researched species in AD have been: *Lactobacillus rhamnosus GG, Bifidobacterium lactis,* and *Streptococcus thermophiles* [74].

One study recruited children aged 4–48 months with atopic dermatitis to evaluate the effects of a *L. rhamnosus* GG probiotic. The study was designed as a randomized placebo controlled trial in which participants were either provided *L. rhamnosus* probiotic or a placebo for 8 weeks. Results revealed an average $-\ 23.20 \pm 15.24$ change in the Scoring of Atopic Dermatitis (SCORAD) score ($p = 0.003$). Another study recruited 38 adult patients with AD and instructed them to either take a probiotic strain *Lactobacillus salivarius* or placebo for 16 weeks [75]. The treatment group also showed significant reductions in the SCORAD score at 16 weeks ($p < 0.001$) and no significant reductions in the control group.

A study conducted in 2010, evaluated the effects of a mixture of two probiotic strains: *Lactobacillus acidophilus* DDS-1 and *Bifidobacterium lactis* UABLA-12 combined with fructo-oligosaccharide [76]. 90 children with moderate to severe AD aged 1–3 years were asked to take the probiotic mixture or control for 8 weeks. Average SCORAD scores decreased more significantly than scores in the placebo group ($p = 0.001$). The study also found significant decreases in CD4 and CD25 counts and increased CD8 counts in the probiotic counts compared to placebo($p < 0.007$) suggesting the use of probiotics in AD may have immunomodulatory effects.

Overall, many studies have displayed the positive effects of probiotics on AD severity. Thus, probiotics provide another treatment modality that patients suffering from AD can use along with traditional treatments.

2.6.2 L-Histidine

As the pathophysiology of AD is complex, one aspect that has been studied is the disruption of the skin barrier. Research has shown that one gene, the filaggrin gene, can be mutated in patients with AD and causes loss of function in the filaggrin protein which normally contributes to the integrity of the epidermis and skin barrier [77]. This has been proposed to cause a predisposition to developing AD in some patients. L-histidine has been suggested to contribute to the formation of the filaggrin protein and thus research has theorized that L-histidine supplementation could improve the skin barrier in AD [78].

One study assessed the effects of L-histidine in both adult and children populations [78]. 24 adults were asked to take either 4 g oral L-histidine or placebo for 8 weeks. A 34% reduction in SCORAD scores was found in the treatment group after 4 weeks ($p < 0.003$). Additionally, 49 children aged 1–7 years with AD were asked to either consume 0.8 g oral L-histidine daily or placebo for 12 weeks. Similarly, the treatment group showed a decrease in SCORAD score by 49% at 12 weeks and placebo had no significant changes ($p < 0.02$).

An additional study in 2017 studied the effects of L-histidine in vivo and in vitro [79]. The in vitro study utilized human keratinocyte cultures to supplement with L-histidine and results indicated increases in filaggrin formation ($p < 0.01$). The clinical study was conducted with 24 adult participants with AD who agreed to a 2 week washout period and use of any other treatments for AD. They were then assigned to either take 4 g of L-histidine (Group A) or placebo (Group B) for the first 8 weeks after which crossover occurred and patients took the opposite intervention for an additional 8 weeks. The results showed that Group A had a 32% decrease in SCORAD scores at week 8 ($P = 0.0029$), however the statistical analysis could not be performed "meaningfully" in Group B after crossover [79]. In conclusion, the literature supports L-histidine supplementation as a beneficial complementary therapy to current standard treatments for AD.

3 Key Takeaways and Summary

Since many inflammatory dermatologic conditions such as acne, psoriasis, HS, AD, and rosacea are very complex and multifactorial, it is vital to take a holistic approach to optimize the management of these conditions and improve overall quality of life from those suffering with these diseases. Immunomodulation is a therapeutic strategy that enhances or suppresses the endogenous immune system for the treatment of various diseases, cancers, and infections. Immunomodulatory agents include prescription drugs such as JAK inhibitors, immune checkpoint inhibitors, PDE-4 inhibitors, and biologics. In addition, nutrition, supplements, topical botanicals, and probiotics have been demonstrated to have immunologic activity, while often lacking the adverse sequelae characteristic of FDA-approved prescription immunomodulators. Thus, it is imperative clinicians provide adequate education and guidance to their patients regarding the additional modalities in which each condition can be managed including nutrition modifications, dietary supplements, and topical options based on the latest supporting research.

Nutrition has a profound impact on the state of disease severity for many dermatologic disorders. Research has shown that certain diets can be extremely beneficial for decreasing disease severity and have immunomodulatory properties. For instance, following a brewer's yeast exclusion diet has shown to decrease skin lesions in HS and any deviations from this diet resulted in recurrence of symptoms [52, 53]. Additionally, a low glycemic diet has shown to decrease acne lesion counts in those with mild to moderate acne [31]. The avoidance of milk, especially skim milk, can be said to be beneficial for those suffering from acne as milk consumption has shown to be correlated to acne exacerbations [19–22].[8, 10] Furthermore, the relation of chocolate to acne is unclear and no strong support is evident for its correlation with acne [23].

Various supplements, probiotics, and herbals have been outlined in the literature as having therapeutic and immunomodulatory effects on many inflammatory conditions. Probiotic use has been most extensively studied for the management of acne vulgaris, although novel research addressing the cutaneous and gastrointestinal microbiome among HS patients suggests probiotic strategies may effectively supplement conventional HS therapies. The efficacy of probiotics for use in acne may be largely due to the inhibition of *C. acnes* growth via the production of bacteriocins [13]; in contrast, probiotics are postulated to be efficacious in the management of HS due to replenishment of *C. acnes*, in addition to *Staphylococcus epidermidis* and *Corynebacterium* spp. [60]. Ultimately, controlled, clinical trials are necessary to validate current hypotheses regarding the role of probiotics in HS. Similarly, the use of probiotics and L-histidine has been well supported by many studies to decrease SCORAD scores in AD [76, 78, 79].

Various supplements have been assessed for the management of HS and psoriasis. Zinc supplementation was first demonstrated to be efficacious in the clearance of HS-associated lesion in 1960 with a case-series including six patients [78]. Furthermore, a 2007 study observed dose-dependent remission with zinc gluconate oral supplementation [56]. Oral zinc and nicotinamide supplements have depicted efficacy as maintenance therapy, depicting the utility of oral supplements in conjunction with conventional therapeutic strategies [57]. Larger, controlled trials are necessary to increase the robustness of results discussed in prior small, observational studies.

Lastly, topical botanicals have been extensively studied for therapeutic management of rosacea and psoriasis. In addition to FDA approved topical treatments for rosacea, botanical therapies and natural products have been assessed for improvement in rosacea-associated facial erythema, papule and pustule counts, and telangiectasia. Facial erythema and papule and pustule counts were most reliably improved by the use of botanical topicals, either in isolation or in conjunction with other therapies, such as cryotherapy. Despite the observed efficacy of *Quassia amara* extract, silymarin and niacinamide cream failed to elicit improvement in the appearance of telangiectasia. Common adverse effects of topical botanical use can include transient burning, pruritus, and even hypersensitivity reactions [63]. Additionally, the use of topical botanicals has been promising for use in psoriasis. Botanicals including aloe vera, indigo naturalis, and *Mahonia aquifolium* have shown to significantly improve psoriatic lesions and improve PASI scores [66].

In conclusion, the treatment of inflammatory dermatologic disorders should be approached through a holistic way. The literature has extensively supported and proven the immunomodulatory effects of nutrition, supplements, probiotics, and botanicals for the treatment of various conditions including HS, AD, acne vulgaris, psoriasis, and rosacea. Thus, moving forward clinicians can provide patients with a variety of choices for treatment optimization.

References

1. Mian M, Silfvast-Kaiser A, Paek S, Kivelevitch D, Menter A. A review of the most common dermatologic conditions and their debilitating psychosocial impacts. Int Arch Internal Med. 2019;3. https://doi.org/10.23937/2643-4466/1710018
2. Bhate K, Williams HC. Epidemiology of acne vulgaris. Br J Dermatol. 2013;168(3):474–85. https://doi.org/10.1111/bjd.12149.
3. Thielitz A, Abdel-Naser MB, Fluhr JW, Zouboulis CC, Gollnick H. Topical retinoids in acne–an evidence-based overview. J Dtsch Dermatol Ges. 2008;6(12):1023–31. https://doi.org/10.1111/j.1610-0387.2008.06741.x.
4. Matin T, Goodman MB. Benzoyl peroxide. In: StatPearls. StatPearls Publishing; 2022. http://www.ncbi.nlm.nih.gov/books/NBK537220/. Accessed 15 Dec 2022
5. Zaenglein AL, Pathy AL, Schlosser BJ, et al. Guidelines of care for the management of acne vulgaris. J Am Acad Dermatol. 2016;74(5):945-973.e33. https://doi.org/10.1016/j.jaad.2015.12.037.
6. Dao M, Kelsberg G, Louden D. Potential harms of long-term acne treatment with oral antibiotics. Can Fam Physician. 2020;66(9):669–70.
7. McLaughlin J, Watterson S, Layton AM, Bjourson AJ, Barnard E, McDowell A. Propionibacterium acnes and acne vulgaris: new insights from the integration of population genetic, multi-omic, biochemical and host-microbe studies. Microorganisms. 2019;7(5):128. https://doi.org/10.3390/microorganisms7050128.
8. Al-Ghazzewi FH, Tester RF. Effect of konjac glucomannan hydrolysates and probiotics on the growth of the skin bacterium Propionibacterium acnes in vitro. Int J Cosmet Sci. 2010;32(2):139–42. https://doi.org/10.1111/j.1468-2494.2009.00555.x.
9. Llewellyn A, Foey A. Probiotic modulation of innate cell pathogen sensing and signaling events. Nutrients. 2017;9(10):1156. https://doi.org/10.3390/nu9101156.
10. Kober MM, Bowe WP. The effect of probiotics on immune regulation, acne, and photoaging. Int J Womens Dermatol. 2015;1(2):85–9. https://doi.org/10.1016/j.ijwd.2015.02.001.
11. Hacini-Rachinel F, Gheit H, Le Luduec JB, Dif F, Nancey S, Kaiserlian D. Oral probiotic control skin inflammation by acting on both effector and regulatory T cells. PLoS ONE. 2009;4(3):e4903. https://doi.org/10.1371/journal.pone.0004903.
12. Bowe WP, Filip JC, DiRienzo JM, Volgina A, Margolis DJ. Inhibition of propionibacterium acnes by bacteriocin-like inhibitory substances (BLIS) produced by Streptococcus salivarius. J Drugs Dermatol. 2006;5(9):868–70.

13. Oh S, Kim SH, Ko Y, et al. Effect of bacteriocin produced by Lactococcus sp. HY 449 on skin-inflammatory bacteria. Food Chem Toxicol. 2006;44(8):1184–90. https://doi.org/10.1016/j.fct.2005.08.008
14. Marchetti F, Capizzi R, Tulli A. Efficacy of regulators of the intestinal bacterial flora in the therapy of acne vulgaris. Clin Ter. 1987;122(5):339–43.
15. Jung GW, Tse JE, Guiha I, Rao J. Prospective, randomized, open-label trial comparing the safety, efficacy, and tolerability of an acne treatment regimen with and without a probiotic supplement and minocycline in subjects with mild to moderate acne. J Cutan Med Surg. 2013;17(2):114–22. https://doi.org/10.2310/7750.2012.12026.
16. Lebeer S, Oerlemans E, Claes I, et al. Topical cream with live lactobacilli modulates the skin microbiome and reduce acne symptoms 2018. https://doi.org/10.1101/463307
17. Kang BS, Seo JG, Lee GS, et al. Antimicrobial activity of enterocins from Enterococcus faecalis SL-5 against Propionibacterium acnes, the causative agent in acne vulgaris, and its therapeutic effect. J Microbiol. 2009;47(1):101–9. https://doi.org/10.1007/s12275-008-0179-y.
18. Muizzuddin N, Maher W, Sullivan M, Schnittger S, Mammone T. Physiological effect of a probiotic on skin. J Cosmet Sci. 2012;63(6):385–95.
19. Melnik BC, Schmitz G. Role of insulin, insulin-like growth factor-1, hyperglycaemic food and milk consumption in the pathogenesis of acne vulgaris. Exp Dermatol. 2009;18(10):833–41. https://doi.org/10.1111/j.1600-0625.2009.00924.x.
20. Juhl CR, Bergholdt HKM, Miller IM, Jemec GBE, Kanters JK, Ellervik C. Dairy intake and acne vulgaris: a systematic review and meta-analysis of 78,529 children, adolescents, and young adults. Nutrients. 2018;10(8):1049. https://doi.org/10.3390/nu10081049.
21. Penso L, Touvier M, Deschasaux M, et al. Association between adult acne and dietary behaviors: findings from the NutriNet-Santé prospective cohort study. JAMA Dermatol. 2020;156(8):854–62. https://doi.org/10.1001/jamadermatol.2020.1602.
22. Adebamowo CA, Spiegelman D, Danby FW, Frazier AL, Willett WC, Holmes MD. High school dietary dairy intake and teenage acne. J Am Acad Dermatol. 2005;52(2):207–14. https://doi.org/10.1016/j.jaad.2004.08.007.
23. Goh W, Kallianpur KJ, Chow D, et al. Chocolate and acne: how valid was the original study? Clin Dermatol. 2011;29(4):459–60. https://doi.org/10.1016/j.clindermatol.2011.05.002.
24. Caperton C, Block S, Viera M, Keri J, Berman B. Double-blind, placebo-controlled study assessing the effect of chocolate consumption in subjects with a history of acne vulgaris. J Clin Aesthet Dermatol. 2014;7(5):19–23.
25. Grant JD, Anderson PC. Chocolate as a cause of acne: a dissenting view. Mo Med. 1965;62:459–60.
26. Fulton JE Jr, Plewig G, Kligman AM. Effect of chocolate on acne vulgaris. JAMA. 1969;210(11):2071–4. https://doi.org/10.1001/jama.1969.03160370055011.
27. Delost GR, Delost ME, Lloyd J. The impact of chocolate consumption on acne vulgaris in college students: a randomized crossover study. J Am Acad Dermatol 2016;75(1):220–2. https://doi.org/10.1016/j.jaad.2016.02.1159
28. Ni C, Jia Q, Ding G, Wu X, Yang M. Low-glycemic index diets as an intervention in metabolic diseases: a systematic review and meta-analysis. Nutrients. 2022;14(2):307. https://doi.org/10.3390/nu14020307.
29. Glycemic index and how it affects your diet. Cleveland Clinic. https://health.clevelandclinic.org/glycemic-index/. Published 21Oct 2021. Accessed 17 Dec 2022.
30. Smith RN, Mann NJ, Braue A, Mäkeläinen H, Varigos GA. A low-glycemic-load diet improves symptoms in acne vulgaris patients: a randomized controlled trial. Am J Clin Nutr. 2007;86(1):107–15. https://doi.org/10.1093/ajcn/86.1.107.
31. Kwon H, Yoon J, Hong J, Jung J, Park M, Suh D. Clinical and histological effect of a low glycaemic load diet in treatment of acne vulgaris in Korean patients: a randomized controlled trial. Acta Derm Venerol. 2012;92(3):241–6. https://doi.org/10.2340/00015555-1346.
32. Armstrong AW, Mehta MD, Schupp CW, Gondo GC, Bell SJ, Griffiths CEM. Psoriasis prevalence in adults in the United States. JAMA Dermatol. 2021;157(8):940–6. https://doi.org/10.1001/jamadermatol.2021.2007.

33. Badri T, Kumar P, Oakley AM. Plaque psoriasis. In: StatPearls. StatPearls Publishing; 2022. http://www.ncbi.nlm.nih.gov/books/NBK430879/. Accessed 16 Dec 2022.
34. Takeshita J, Grewal S, Langan SM, et al. Psoriasis and comorbid diseases. J Am Acad Dermatol. 2017;76(3):377–90. https://doi.org/10.1016/j.jaad.2016.07.064.
35. Zhou X, Chen Y, Cui L, Shi Y, Guo C. Advances in the pathogenesis of psoriasis: from keratinocyte perspective. Cell Death Dis. 2022;13(1):1–13. https://doi.org/10.1038/s41419-022-04523-3.
36. Hawkes JE, Chan TC, Krueger JG. Psoriasis pathogenesis and the development of novel targeted immune therapies. J Allergy Clin Immunol. 2017;140(3):645–53. https://doi.org/10.1016/j.jaci.2017.07.004.
37. Armstrong AW, Read C. Pathophysiology, clinical presentation, and treatment of psoriasis: a review. JAMA. 2020;323(19):1945–60. https://doi.org/10.1001/jama.2020.4006.
38. Pona A, Haidari W, Kolli SS, Feldman SR. Diet and psoriasis. Dermatol Online J. 2019;25(2):13030/qt1p37435s.
39. Jensen P, Zachariae C, Christensen R, et al. Effect of weight loss on the severity of psoriasis: a randomized clinical study. JAMA Dermatol. 2013;149(7):795–801. https://doi.org/10.1001/jamadermatol.2013.722
40. Al-Mutairi N, Nour T. The effect of weight reduction on treatment outcomes in obese patients with psoriasis on biologic therapy: a randomized controlled prospective trial. Expert Opin Biol Ther. 2014;14(6):749–56. https://doi.org/10.1517/14712598.2014.900541
41. Gisondi P, Del Giglio M, Di Francesco V, Zamboni M, Girolomoni G. Weight loss improves the response of obese patients with moderate-to-severe chronic plaque psoriasis to low-dose cyclosporine therapy: a randomized, controlled, investigator-blinded clinical trial. Am J Clin Nutr. 2008;88(5):1242–47. https://doi.org/10.3945/ajcn.2008.26427
42. Artemniak-Wojtowicz D, Kucharska AM, Pyrżak B. Obesity and chronic inflammation crosslinking. Cent Eur J Immunol. 2020;45(4):461–68. https://doi.org/10.5114/ceji.2020.103418
43. Mayser P, Mrowietz U, Arenberger P, et al. Omega-3 fatty acid-based lipid infusion in patients with chronic plaque psoriasis: results of a double-blind, randomized, placebo-controlled, multicenter trial. J Am Acad Dermatol. 1998;38(4):539–47. https://doi.org/10.1016/s0190-9622(98)70114-8
44. Lassus A, Dahlgren AL, Halpern MJ, Santalahti J, Happonen HP. Effects of dietary supplementation with polyunsaturated ethyl ester lipids (Angiosan) in patients with psoriasis and psoriatic arthritis. J Int Med Res. 1990;18(1):68–73. https://doi.org/10.1177/030006059001800109
45. Gupta AK, Ellis CN, Goldfarb MT, Hamilton TA, Voorhees JJ. The role of fish oil in psoriasis. A randomized, double-blind, placebo-controlled study to evaluate the effect of fish oil and topical corticosteroid therapy in psoriasis. Int J Dermatol. 1990;29(8):591–95. https://doi.org/10.1111/j.1365-4362.1990.tb03477.x
46. Farahnik B, Sharma D, Alban J, Sivamani RK. Topical botanical agents for the treatment of psoriasis: a systematic review. Am J Clin Dermatol. 2017;18(4):451–68. https://doi.org/10.1007/s40257-017-0266-0
47. Augustin M, Andrees U, Grimme H, Schöpf E, Simon J. Effects of *Mahonia aquifolium* ointment on the expression of adhesion, proliferation, and activation markers in the skin of patients with psoriasis. Forsch Komplementarmed. 1999;6 Suppl 2:19–21. https://doi.org/10.1159/000057142
48. Lin YK, See LC, Huang YH, et al. Comparison of refined and crude indigo naturalis ointment in treating psoriasis: randomized, observer-blind, controlled, intrapatient trial. Arch Dermatol. 2012;148(3):397–400. https://doi.org/10.1001/archdermatol.2011.1091
49. Syed TA, Ahmad SA, Holt AH, Ahmad SA, Ahmad SH, Afzal M. Management of psoriasis with Aloe vera extract in a hydrophilic cream: a placebo-controlled, double-blind study. Trop Med Int Health. 1996;1(4):505–09. https://doi.org/10.1046/j.1365-3156.1996.d01-91.x
50. Nesbitt E, Clements S, Driscoll M. A concise clinician's guide to therapy for hidradenitis suppurativa. Int J Womens Dermatol. 2019;6(2):80–4. https://doi.org/10.1016/j.ijwd.2019.11.004.

51. van Straalen KR. Anti-Saccharomyces cerevisiae antibodies could reflect distinct phenotypes in hidradenitis suppurativa. J Allergy Clin Immunol. 2020;146(2):461. https://doi.org/10.1016/j.jaci.2020.04.017.
52. Cannistrà C, Finocchi V, Trivisonno A, Tambasco D. New perspectives in the treatment of hidradenitis suppurativa: surgery and brewer's yeast–exclusion diet. Surgery. 2013;154(5):1126–30. https://doi.org/10.1016/j.surg.2013.04.018.
53. Aboud C, Zamaria N, Cannistrà C. Treatment of hidradenitis suppurativa: Surgery and yeast (Saccharomyces cerevisiae)–exclusion diet. Results after 6 years. Surgery. 2020;167(6):1012–5. https://doi.org/10.1016/j.surg.2019.12.015
54. Sivanand A, Gulliver WP, Josan CK, Alhusayen R, Fleming PJ. Weight loss and dietary interventions for hidradenitis suppurativa: a systematic review. J Cutan Med Surg. 2020;24(1):64–72. https://doi.org/10.1177/1203475419874412.
55. Mackenna RM, Lehmann H. The glucose tolerance curve in hidradenitis suppurativa. Br J Dermatol. 1960;72:142–4. https://doi.org/10.1111/j.1365-2133.1960.tb13862.x.
56. Brocard A, Knol AC, Khammari A, Dréno B. Hidradenitis suppurativa and zinc: a new therapeutic approach. A pilot study. Dermatology. 2007;214(4):325–7. https://doi.org/10.1159/000100883.
57. Molinelli E, Brisigotti V, Campanati A, et al. Efficacy of oral zinc and nicotinamide as maintenance therapy for mild/moderate hidradenitis suppurativa: a controlled retrospective clinical study. J Am Acad Dermatol. 2020;83(2):665–7. https://doi.org/10.1016/j.jaad.2020.04.092.
58. Guillet A, Brocard A, Bach Ngohou K, et al. Verneuil's disease, innate immunity and vitamin D: a pilot study. J Eur Acad Dermatol Venereol. 2015;29(7):1347–53. https://doi.org/10.1111/jdv.12857.
59. Frew JW. Hidradenitis suppurativa is an autoinflammatory keratinization disease: a review of the clinical, histologic, and molecular evidence. JAAD Int. 2020;1(1):62–72. https://doi.org/10.1016/j.jdin.2020.05.005.
60. Ring HC, Thorsen J, Fuursted K, et al. Probiotics in hidradenitis suppurativa: a potential treatment option? Clin Exp Dermatol. 2022;47(1):139–41. https://doi.org/10.1111/ced.14838.
61. Wark KJL, Cains GD. The microbiome in hidradenitis suppurativa: a review. Dermatol Ther (Heidelberg). 2021;11(1):39–52. https://doi.org/10.1007/s13555-020-00465-w.
62. Ring HC, Thorsen J, Jørgensen AH, et al. Predictive metagenomic analysis reveals a role of cutaneous dysbiosis in the development of hidradenitis suppurativa. J Invest Dermatol. 2020;140(7):1473–6. https://doi.org/10.1016/j.jid.2019.11.011.
63. Fisk WA, Lev-Tov HA, Clark AK, Sivamani RK. Phytochemical and botanical therapies for rosacea: a systematic review. Phytother Res. 2015;29(10):1439–51. https://doi.org/10.1002/ptr.5432.
64. Gether L, Overgaard LK, Egeberg A, Thyssen JP. Incidence and prevalence of rosacea: a systematic review and meta-analysis. Br J Dermatol. 2018;179(2):282–9. https://doi.org/10.1111/bjd.16481.
65. Rainer BM, Kang S, Chien AL. Rosacea: epidemiology, pathogenesis, and treatment. Dermatoendocrinology. 2017;9(1): e1361574. https://doi.org/10.1080/19381980.2017.1361574.
66. Rigopoulos D, Kalogeromitros D, Gregoriou S, et al. Randomized placebo-controlled trial of a flavonoid-rich plant extract-based cream in the treatment of rosacea. J Eur Acad Dermatol Venereol. 2005;19(5):564–8. https://doi.org/10.1111/j.1468-3083.2005.01248.x.
67. Ferrari A, Diehl C. Evaluation of the efficacy and tolerance of a topical gel with 4% quassia extract in the treatment of rosacea. J Clin Pharmacol. 2012;52(1):84–8. https://doi.org/10.1177/0091270010391533.
68. Broniarczyk-Dyła G, Prusińska-Bratoś M, Kmieć ML. Assessment of the influence of licochalcone on selected functional skin parameters in patients with impaired vasomotor disorders and rosacea. Adv Dermatol Allergology/Postępy Dermatologii i Alergologii. 2011;28(4):241–7.
69. Weber TM, Ceilley RI, Buerger A, et al. Skin tolerance, efficacy, and quality of life of patients with red facial skin using a skin care regimen containing Licochalcone A. J Cosmet Dermatol. 2006;5(3):227–32. https://doi.org/10.1111/j.1473-2165.2006.00261.x

70. Yu TG, Zheng YZ, Zhu JT, Guo W. Effect of treatment of rosacea in females by Chibixiao Recipe (赤鼻消方) in combination with minocycline and spironolactone. Chin J Integr Med 2006;12(4):277–80. https://doi.org/10.1007/s11655-006-0277-1
71. Kapur S, Watson W, Carr S. Atopic dermatitis. Allergy asthma. Clin Immunol. 2018;14(Suppl 2):52. https://doi.org/10.1186/s13223-018-0281-6.
72. David Boothe W, Tarbox JA, Tarbox MB. Atopic dermatitis: pathophysiology. In: Fortson EA, Feldman SR, Strowd LC, editors. Management of atopic dermatitis: methods and challenges. Advances in experimental medicine and biology. Springer International Publishing;2017. p. 21–37. https://doi.org/10.1007/978-3-319-64804-0_3
73. Frazier W, Bhardwaj N. Atopic dermatitis: diagnosis and treatment. AFP. 2020;101(10):590–8.
74. Schlichte MJ, Vandersall A, Katta R. Diet and eczema: a review of dietary supplements for the treatment of atopic dermatitis. Dermatol Pract Concept. 2016;6(3):23–9. https://doi.org/10.5826/dpc.0603a06.
75. Drago L, Iemoli E, Rodighiero V, Nicola L, De Vecchi E, Piconi S. Effects of lactobacillus salivarius LS01 (DSM 22775) treatment on adult atopic dermatitis: a randomized placebo-controlled study. Int J Immunopathol Pharmacol. 2011;24(4):1037–48. https://doi.org/10.1177/039463201102400421.
76. Gerasimov S, Vasjuta V, Myhovych O, Bondarchuk L. Probiotic supplement reduces atopic dermatitis in preschool children: a randomized, double-blind, placebo-controlled, clinical trial. Am J Clin Dermatol. 2010;11:351–61. https://doi.org/10.2165/11531420-000000000-00000.
77. Osawa R, Akiyama M, Shimizu H. Filaggrin gene defects and the risk of developing allergic disorders. Allergol Int. 2011;60(1):1–9. https://doi.org/10.2332/allergolint.10-RAI-0270.
78. Gibbs NK. L-histidine supplementation in adults and young children with atopic dermatitis (Eczema). J Nutr. 2020;150(Suppl 1):2576S-2579S. https://doi.org/10.1093/jn/nxaa200.
79. Tan SP, Brown SB, Griffiths CE, Weller RB, Gibbs NK. Feeding filaggrin: effects of l-histidine supplementation in atopic dermatitis. Clin Cosmet Investig Dermatol. 2017;10:403–11. https://doi.org/10.2147/CCID.S146760.

Immunomodulators and Biologics for Follicular and Neutrophilic Cutaneous Disorders

Mavra Masood and Iltefat Hamzavi

Abstract There are several different immunomodulatory and biologic therapies used in the treatment of moderate to severe hidradenitis suppurativa, cutaneous vasculitis, and pyoderma gangrenosum. Selection of therapy is dependent on severity of disease. There is evidence that suggests continuation of biologic therapy while pursuing surgical treatment of HS lesions is safe and efficacious. Further studies are needed on the dosing and response of JAK inhibitors for treatment of HS. Biologic therapies are indicated for relapsing pyoderma gangrenosum and cutaneous vasculitis. Future studies examining biologic targets and molecules are underway and will propel treatments to become more targeted in nature for these inflammatory diseases.

Keywords Immunomodulators · Biologic medications · Small molecule inhibitors · Hidradenitis suppurativa · Vasculitis · Pyoderma gangrenosum

1 Introduction

The use of biologics and immunomodulators is an expansive field with many applications in dermatology. In the past 10 years, the presence of different biologic medications has skyrocketed as targeted therapies become available. This chapter will go over the pathophysiology of HS, different biologic and small molecule inhibitor treatments available along with safety and dosing information as well as current treatment guidelines, lab monitoring, and perspectives on surgery with biologics. We will also cover treatment options available for pyoderma gangrenosum and cutaneous vasculitis.

M. Masood · I. Hamzavi (✉)
Department of Dermatology, Henry Ford Hospital, Detroit, MI, USA
e-mail: IHamzavi@hamzavi.com
URL: https://www.Hamzaviderm.com

I. Hamzavi
Department of Dermatology, Henry Ford Hospital, Wayne State University, Detroit, MI, USA

N. Bhatia (ed.), *Immunomodulators and Biologics in Dermatologic Treatment*,
https://doi.org/10.1007/978-3-031-66590-5_10

2 Hidradenitis Suppurativa

Hidradenitis Suppurative (HS) is a chronic recurring inflammatory disease affecting apocrine gland bearing skin [1]. It is characterized by the development of inflammatory and nodules, sinus tracts, fistulae, and scarring which all have significant impacts on quality of life [1]. Treatment modalities often require a multimodal approach as once patients reach Hurley Stage II-III, they should be considered for an immunomodulatory agent. At this point, the patient has already developed at least sinus tunnel and scarring within a region which prompts for greater procedural management as well as optimized medical management. There are several biologic medications and immunomodulatory agents that may be of use however much remains to be investigated.

3 Immune Dysregulation in Hidradenitis Suppurativa

The pathophysiology of HS is not fully understood and the pathogenesis of HS is thought to be due to immune dysregulation and cytokine expression. There is occlusion of the upper part of the hair follicle which lead to perifollicular lymphohistiocytic inflammation [2]. This leads to recruitment of neutrophils, macrophages, monocytes and dendritic cells. Toll like receptor 2 (TLR-2) is highly expressed in by macrophages and dendritic cells, along with IL-12 and IL-23 by macrophages. IL-23 involves the induction of T helper cells (Th17) which is skewed towards production of IL-17 [3].

There is overexpression of IL-1beta, CYCL9 (MIG), IL-10, IL-11, and BLC while IL-20 and IL-22 are downregulated [3]. There is also a component of an inappropriate immune response to bacteria flora and biofilms on the skin, which is further supported by the increase in TLR2 on antigen presenting cells [4]. There may be an interplay with IL-26 and decreased skin amicrobial activity [5]. While several proinflammatory cytokines are implicated in the development of HS, there are limited options in biologic medications targeting these cytokines.

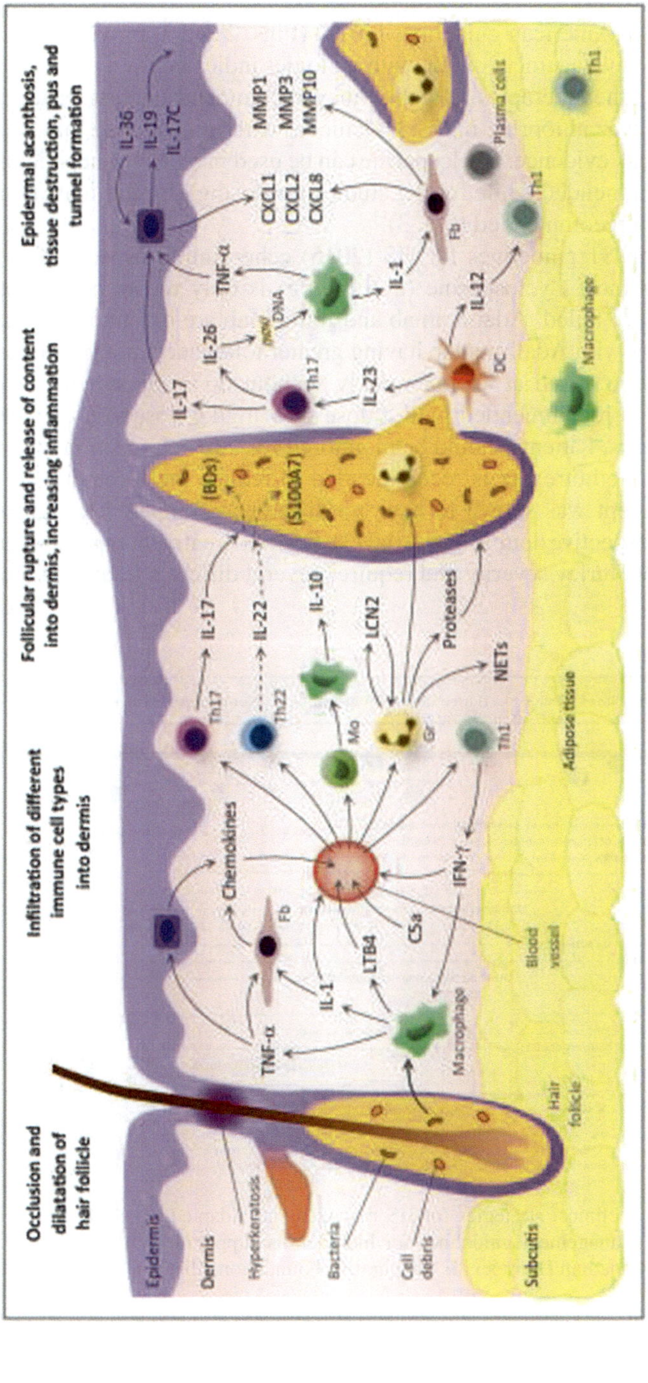

Fig. 1 Pathogenetic events in HS. Adapted from aetiology and pathogenesis of hidradenitis suppurativa. Wolk et al. [2]

4 Current Guidelines

The current North American guidelines (2019) (Figs. 2 and 3) provide a therapeutic algorithm for the management of HS, with biologics indicated for moderate to severe HS along with other therapies. Notably, they recommend against treatment with methotrexate and azathioprine in HS. Colchicine with minocycline may be recommended with weak evidence. Cyclosporine can be used in recalcitrant patients. Adalimumab is recommended while further studies for dosing of infliximab are needed. Etanercept is not recommended (Fig. 3).

The European S1 guidelines for HS (2015) echo similar aspects of the North American guidelines. Cyclosporine (2–6 mg/kg) is only recommended after 3rd line therapies have failed. Adalimumab and Infliximab are recommended based on current evidence, with Adalimumab having greater tolerance among patients. Adalimumab should be dosed at 40 mg weekly without dose adjustment for obesity. Infliximab is also recommended with a dose of 5 mg/kg dosed on day zero, 2, 6 then every 8 weeks. Patients should be monitored for infusion reaction with the first administration. Methotrexate is recommended to reduce the formation of autoantibodies. Etanercept was shown to have no difference compared to placebo after 3 months in a prospective double blind trial [3]. Overall, treatment is recommended by determination of Hurley severity and requires several different treatment modalities (Fig. 4).

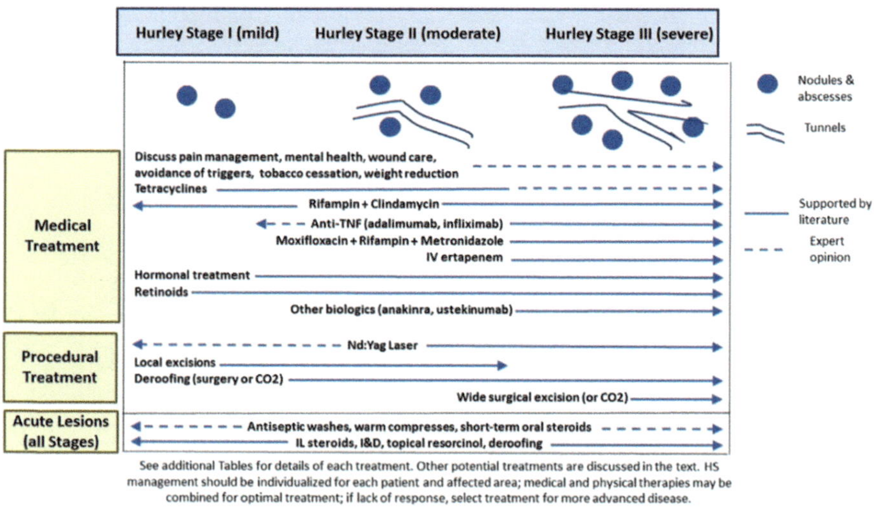

Fig. 2 Overview of clinical strategies for HS management. Adapted from Alikhan et al. North American clinical management guidelines for hidradenitis suppurativa: A publication from the United States and Canadian Hidradenitis Suppurativa Foundations [5]

Recommendations for biologics
Adalimumab at the approved HS dosing is recommended to improve disease severity and quality of life in patients with moderate-to-severe HS.
Infliximab is recommended for moderate-to-severe disease; however, dose-ranging studies are needed to determine the optimal dosage for management.
Anakinra, 100 mg daily, may be effective for HS; however, dose-ranging studies are needed to determine the optimal dosage for management.
Ustekinumab, 45 to 90 mg administered every 12 weeks, may be effective for HS; however, placebo-controlled dose-ranging studies are needed to determine the optimal dosage for management.
The limited available evidence does not support etanercept for the management of HS.

HS, Hidradenitis suppurativa.

Fig. 3 Table of biologic recommendations. Adapted from Alikhan et al. North American clinical management guidelines for hidradenitis suppurativa: A publication from the United States and Canadian Hidradenitis Suppurativa Foundations [5]

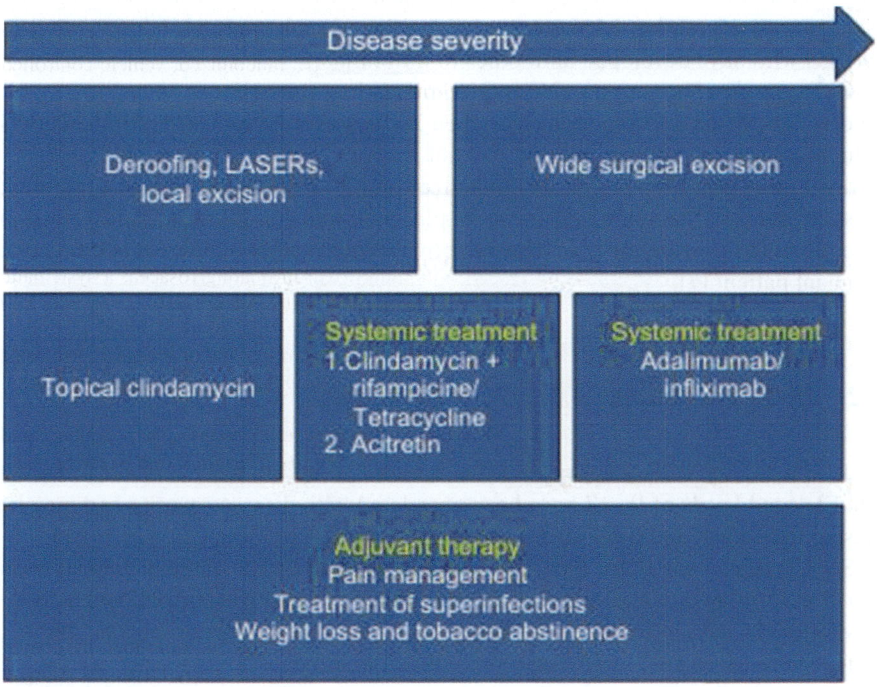

Fig. 4 HS treatment ladder. Adapted from European S1 HS management guidelines. European S1 guideline for the treatment of hidradenitis suppurativa/acne inversa [3]

5 Biologic Medications

5.1 *Anti-TNF Biologics*

Tumor Necrosis Factor (TNF) is a cytokine that is proinflammatory and upregulated in HS lesional skin [1].

Adalimumab is a human IgG1 antibody and is the only FDA approved biologic agent for HS, obtaining around a 50% therapeutic response in patients [6]. It remains the only biologic with a grade A recommendation by the North American clinical guidelines [5]. It is dosed from 160 mg on day 0, 160 mg on week 2, then 40 mg weekly. It is generally well tolerated among patients and should be started early as a delay was associated with a decreased clinical response in a multicenter cohort study, suggesting that there is a "window of opportunity" in HS with starting biologic medications[7]. There is also a concern of paradoxical reaction with the use of anti-TNF inhibitors [8].

Infliximab is a chimeric mouse-human antibody against TNF which leads to decreased disease activity. It is dosed based on weight and is traditionally dosed at 5 mg/kg every two weeks and may be escalated. There should be special considerations for obese patients to reach effective dosing which may be at 7.5 mg/kg with escalation to 10 mg/kg. Methotrexate (7.5–10 mg/week) may be administered in patients who have developed antibodies to infliximab.

Golimumab, a human anti-TNF IgG1 antibody has shown improvement in a 2 case reports. It is dosed at 200 mg on day 0 then 100 mg every 4 weeks [1]. Etanercept is a dimeric human TNF receptor but has not shown clinical improvement in HS [1]. Certolizumab pegol is a pegylated humanized anti TNF antibody without a fragment crystallizable (Fc) region which prevents placental transfer. It has been described in case reports to provide relief of disease activity in refractory patients, including one pregnant patient [7].

5.2 *IL-17 Inhibitors*

IL-17 is a highly inflammatory cytokine which is found to have elevated levels in HS. Elevated levels of IL-17 have been correlated with disease severity and may be present in lesional and perilesional skin [1].

Secukinumab was FDA approved for the treatment of HS in June 2023. It is an anti-IL-17a monoclonal antibody and was found to have 70% of patients achieve HiSCR by 24 weeks in an open label trial [7]. In a retrospective cohort study, 2 patients developed IBD after 3 and 5 months of treatment [7]. It is dosed at 300 mg weekly for the first four weeks, then 300 mg every 4 weeks from week 8. It has been approved by the European Medicines Agency (EMA) for the treatment of HS.

There are also ongoing clinical trials for CJM112 which is a fully human monoclonal antibody which blocks the binding of IL17A/F to its receptor [7]. In a meta-analysis, bimekizumab and adalimumab were found to be better agents for the improvement of HiSCR and DLQI compared to secukinumab 300 mg q4w and 300 mg q2w [9]. Brodalumab is a human IgG2 antibody and was shown in 2 open label trials to lead to HiSCR in 100% of patients [7, 10]. It was dosed at 210 mg at day 0, week 1, and week 2 then every other week. It is undergoing further clinical trials.

Bimekizumab is a monoclonal IgG antibody that selectively inhibits IL-17A and 17F. Following a phase II clinical trial, it was found that bimekizumab lead to clinically meaningful improvement with 46% of patients achieving $HiSCR_{75}$ after 12 weeks [11]. In a meta-analysis of 16 RCTs of biologics and small molecule inhibitors, bimekizumab, along with adalimumab, was found to lead to a significant improvement in HiSCR with an acceptable profile [12].

Ixekizumab is a humanized IgG4 antibody against IL-17A and IL-17A/F that has been used in case reports with patients with concomitant psoriasis[7].

There is a risk for the development of inflammatory bowel disease with the use of anti-IL-17 inhibitors and patients should be counseled and screened appropriately before starting medication [7].

5.3 IL-12 and 23 Inhibitors

IL-23 is associated with the development of autoimmunity, and is expressed in humans with autoimmune diseases [1]. Activated macrophages in HS express increased IL-12 and IL-23. Ustekinumab is an agent which binds to the p40 subunit of IL-12 and IL-23 and has been shown to lead to clinical improvement of the Sartorius score after 40 weeks in 82% of patients in a prospective trial [1, 7]. In a cohort study, it was shown that adalimumab, infliximab and ustekinumab all had comparable drug survival [13].

Much is yet to be studied regarding IL-23 therapeutics. Risankizumab has data from one phase II trial showing HiSCR achieved at 16 weeks in 46.8% of patients [7]. Guselkumab is an IgG1-kappa human antibody which neutralizes the p19 unit of Il-23. It has been studied in case series and one phase II clinical trial with 50.8% of patients achieving HiSCR in 16 weeks. It was dosed as 200 mg every 4 weeks as an infusion [7].

5.4 IL-1 Inhibitors

IL-1 is a mediator of local and systemic inflammation by upregulating the production of inflammatory cytokines and cells. IL-1B and TNF-a are-upregulated in lesional HS skin [1].

Anakinra is a recombinant IL-1A and IL-1B receptor antagonist which has shown clinical efficacy of up to 80% in patients in a randomized control trial [1]. However there have been reports of rapid rebound following drug cessation [7]. It is dosed at 100 mg daily subcutaneously.

Canakinumab is a humanized IL-1B antagonist and was shown to improve disease in case studies [7]. Bermekimab is a human recombinant anti IL-alpha antibody which has undergone phase II clinical trials [7]. It is dosed at 7.5 mg/kg every other week via infusion. [7].

5.5 Other Inhibitors

Apremilast is a phosphodiesterase 4 inhibitor used in the treatment of psoriatic arthritis and plaque psoriasis. It limits the production of TNF-a, IL-12, and IL-23 to prevent further inflammation. It is dosed as 30 mg twice daily orally [7]. There are limited trials testing its efficacy in HS [1].

Vilobelimab (IFX-1) is an anti C5a antibody that underwent an open label trial and phase II clinical trials [7]. Avacopan is a C5a receptor antagonist undergoing trials.

CD-20 may be upregulated in chronic HS lesions [14]. Rituximab is a chimeric antibody against CD-20 protein. It has been used in case reports for HS but there is limited data [7]. There are trials underway for Iscalimab, a human antibody against CD-40.

Spesolimab is an IL-36 inhibitor undergoing phase II clinical trials. RGRN-30 is a heat shock protein 90 inhibitor and in a proof-of-concept clinical trial was found to lead to HiSCR-50 in 60% of patients in 16 weeks [15]. HSP90 is a molecular chaperone protein which promotes the activity of proinflammatory proteins.

There are also investigations underway for IL-36R antibody (Imisdolimab), leukotriene inhibitors, and chemokine receptors [7].

6 Small Molecule Inhibitors

6.1 JAK Inhibitors

Janus Kinase (JAK) inhibitors work on four proteins JAK1, JAK2, JAK3, TYK2 which lead to the activation of transcription factors such as signal transducer and transcription activation (STAT) to modulate the inflammatory process [8]. JAKs are activated by signals from the IL-2, IL-4, IL-5, IL-6, IL-13 receptors and type 1 interferons.

Tofacitinib and baricitinib have been tested and lead to improvement in recalcitrant patients however further studies are needed [1]. There are also concerns with safety and increased risk for venous thromboembolism and major adverse cardiovascular events with tofacitinib, baricitinib, and upadacitinib, prompting a black box warning for such. INCB054707 underwent two phase II clinical trials with different doses and 80% of patients who received 30–60 mg of the drug experienced grade 1–2 adverse events. Further studies are needed to evaluate the efficacy and safety [7]. Povorcitinib have also been tested [7].

Upadacitinib is a selective oral JAK-1 inhibitor that has underwent phase II clinical trials and showed that 75% of patients achieved HiSCR at week 4 with up to 100% at week 12 [8].

Brepocitinib is a dual JAK1 and TYK2 inhibitor and with initial trials reporting an improved clinical response [16]. Side effects of JAK inhibitors were most commonly infections, skin disorders, and GI infections [16].

6.2 Other Immunomodulators

Methotrexate is a folate antimetabolite which prevents DNA synthesis. It is not commonly used and is not recommended by the North American clinical guidelines for HS. Cyclosporine is a calcineurin inhibitor which decreases expression of inflammatory cytokines and T cells. There are limited case reports showing treatment with 2-6 mg daily but further trials are needed.

7 Special Populations

7.1 Pediatric

Adalimumab has been approved for use in pediatric patients with HS greater than 12 years old. Commonly reported side effects are injection site reaction, headache, upper respiratory tract infection, and myalgias which are similar to the adult side effect profile [17]. Dosing is weight dependent. Patients who are between 30 and 60 kg may start with 80 mg weekly for 1 week then 40 mg every two weeks. Patients greater than 60 kg should start with 160 mg on day 1 then 80 mg on day 15 with 40 mg weekly after day 29 [17].

Laboratory testing prior to initiation of biologics includes baseline CBC, CMP, TB testing, GGT, Hepatitis panel, and vaccine status for pediatric patients. Children are recommended to be up to date on all immunizations before starting a biologic medication. Live vaccines are not recommended while on a biologic agent due to the risk of inadequate vaccine response and risk for infection.

When vaccines are required, the biologic is recommended to be stopped for at least 3 months prior to vaccination, then reintroduced 2–4 weeks after administration. Patients are able to receive non-live vaccines while on biologic therapy.

It is useful to optimize practical considerations for children prior to biologic delivery. Such measures include using a thinner needle, applying topical anesthetics prior to administration, and making sure the drug is room temperature [17]. The biologic agent should be held when there is a concern for infection.

7.2 Pregnancy

Certolizumab is a PEGylated TNF-alpha inhibitor that is often first line when considering a TNF-alpha blocker. This is due to the inability of the drug to cross the placenta. Based on a physician survey, 59% of physician participants from HS centers had continued the use or prescribed biologics during pregnancy [18, 19]. Immunosuppressive agents should be avoided in pregnant patients.

8 Laboratory Testing

8.1 Screening

There is a risk of reactivation of tuberculosis, HIV, hepatitis B or C, as well as increased risk of infections, myelosuppression and hepatotoxicity with the use of immunomodulatory biologic agents [20]. As a result, most professional societies and the FDA recommend screening patients for the following conditions prior to starting a biologic agent to obtain baseline levels (Figs. 5 and 6). Any patient initiating a TNF-a blocker should undergo screening for tuberculosis. If the test is positive it is recommended to start prophylaxis with isoniazid [21].

Before starting a JAK inhibitor, it is recommended to undergo a CBC with differential, CMP, testing for hepatitis B and C, HIV, lipid panel, and TB [12]. A thorough risk assessment should be conducted to assess if the patient has any coagulation disorder, cardiovascular disease, history of VTE, or malignancy. If possible, patients should be counselled to obtain any pneumococcal or Shingrex vaccine (Fig. 7).

8.2 Monitoring

It is important to continue to monitor patients for anemias and cytopenias once patients are on a TNF blocker. It is recommended to have regular complete blood cell counts every 3–6 months. While TNF blockers are not known to cause hepatotoxicity, there is a risk for increased LFTs on infliximab. Patients with higher risk factors for liver injury may be screened at more frequent intervals [21] (Figs. 5 and 6).

	TB		Hepatitis Panel		CBC		LFT		Lipid Panel	
	Prior	Ongoing	Prior	Ongoing	Prior	Ongoing	Prior	Ongoing	Prior	Ongoing
IL-1 (Anakinra)	Y	-	Y	-	Y	Y	-	-	-	-
Methotrexate	If high risk	-	If high risk	-	Y	Y	Y	Y	-	-
TNFi	Y	If high risk	Y	If carrier	Y	-	Y	Y* Infliximab only	-	-
IL-12/-23i (Ustekinumab)	Y	If high risk	Y	-	Y	Optional	Y	Optional	-	-
IL-23i	Y	If high risk	Y	Y	Y	-	Y	-	-	-
IL-17Ai	Y	If high risk	Y	-	Y	-	Y	-	-	-
IL-4/13i (Dupilumab)	None									
PDE-4i (Apremilast)	None									

Abbreviations: *TNFi*, Tumor necrosis factor inhibitor; *IL*, interleukin; *PDE-4i*, phosphodiesterase-4 inhibitor; *TB*, tuberculosis test; *CBC*, complete blood count; *LFT*, liver function tests; *Y*, yes (recommended), *dash*, no recommendation. Recommendations based on the Joint American Academy of Dermatology-National Psoriasis Foundation guidelines of care. Recommendations for IL-4/13i are from the EuroGuiDerm Centre for Guideline Development. Recommendations for IL-1 are from the American College of Rheumatology Medication Guide.

Fig. 5 Laboratory monitoring guidelines from professional societies. Adapted from prevalence of pre-treatment testing recommended for patients with chronic inflammatory skin diseases [20, 22]

For JAK inhibitors, patients should be monitored 1 month after treatment and obtain a CBC with differential, a CMP, and liver function tests. These tests should be continued every 3 to 6 months with a lipid panel assessed 3 months after initiation. TB Screening should occur annually [23] (Fig. 7).

	TB		Hepatitis Panel		CBC		LFT		Lipid Panel	
	Prior	Ongoing	Prior	Ongoing	Prior	Ongoing	Prior	Ongoing	Prior	Ongoing
IL-1 (Anakinra)	Y	-	Y	-	Y	Y	-	-	-	-
Methotrexate	-	-	-	-	Y	Y	Y	Y	-	-
TNFi	Y	Y	Y	If carrier	-	-	-	-	-	-
IL-12/-23i (Ustekinumab)	Y	-	-	-	-	-	-	-	-	-
IL-23i	Y	-	-	-	-	-	-	-	-	-
IL-17Ai	Y	-	-	-	-	-	-	-	-	-
IL-4/13i (Dupilumab)	None									
PDE-4i (Apremilast)	None									

Abbreviations: *TNFi*, Tumor necrosis factor inhibitor; *IL*, interleukin; *PDE-4i*, phosphodiesterase-4 inhibitor; *TB*, tuberculosis test; *CBC*, complete blood count; *LFT*, liver function tests; *Y*, yes (recommended), *dash*, no recommendation.

Fig. 6 FDA laboratory monitoring guidelines. Adapted from prevalence of pre-treatment testing recommended for patients with chronic inflammatory skin diseases [20, 24]

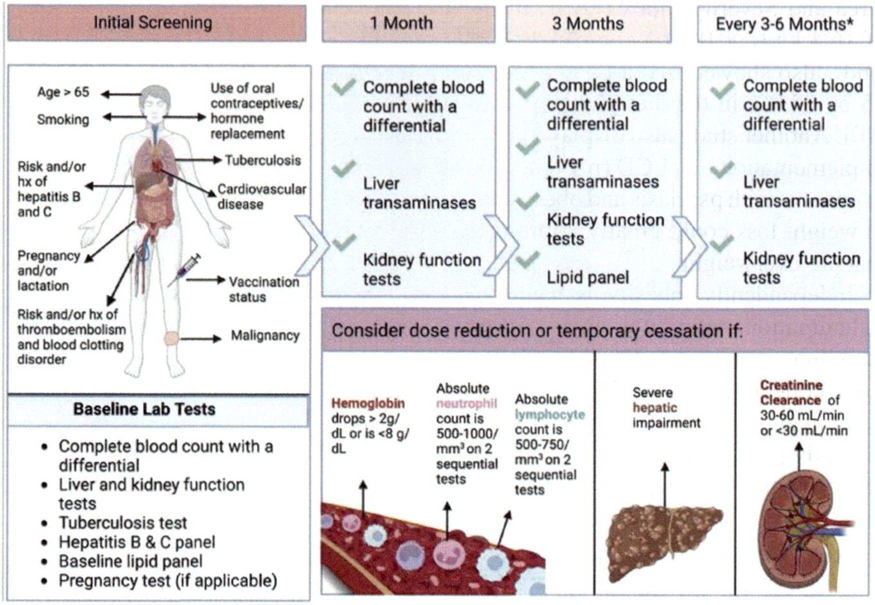

Fig. 7 Screening and laboratory monitoring guidelines for JAK inhibitors. Adapted from a review on the safety of using JAK Inhibitors in Dermatology: Clinical and Laboratory Monitoring [23]

9 Surgery and Biologics

HS requires multimodal treatment with medications to target inflammation while also using surgical and procedural modalities to address scarring and sinus tunnel formation. Post-surgical recurrence can occur in up to 70% of patients depending on the site and procedure performed. This indicates a need for simultaneous anti-inflammatory treatment in conjunction with surgery (Fig. 8).

The SHARPS study was a randomized control trial examining the use of adalimumab in conjunction with surgery. It demonstrated that continuing adalimumab in the perioperative and postoperative period was a safe and effective adjunctive therapy, with no increased risk of postoperative wound infection or complication [26]. In fact, continuing adalimumab for 12 weeks decreased the inflammatory load and reduced HS lesions prior to surgery [26]. A retrospective review was conducted examining the recurrence rate of HS following carbon dioxide laser excision on biologic medications compared to biologic naïve patients [27]. This study found no significant difference in the rate of recurrence between the biologic group (25%) compared to the biologic-naïve group (28%) [27]. Disease progression was observed at a lower rate in the biologic group.

These two studies highlight the safety and efficacy of biologic medications as a mainstay in the treatment of moderate to severe HS along with surgery without affecting surgical outcomes or recurrence rate. As such, biologic treatments should

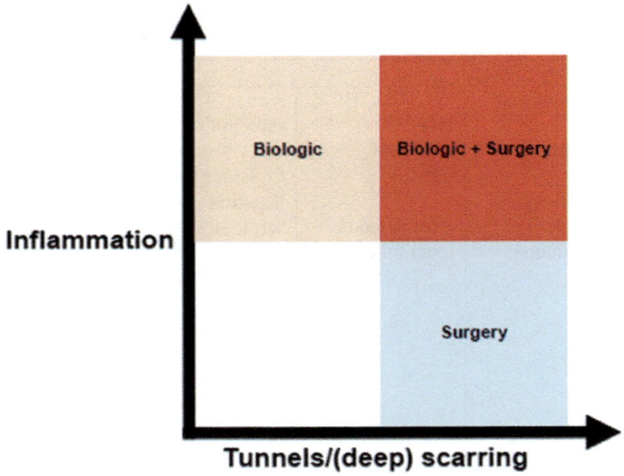

Fig. 8 Combining biologic therapy with surgery. Adapted from clinical implementation of biologics and small molecules in the treatment of hidradenitis suppurativa [25]

aim to be continued using shared decision making between dermatologists and their patients while patients undergo surgical procedures.

10 Future Directions

There are new immunological targets being explored for the treatment of HS. One pathway being explored is potential targeting of CXCR-1 and CXCR-2, which are surface receptors on leukocytes that recruit neutrophils. IL-36 cytokines are part of the IL-1 superfamily and promote inflammation. HS lesional skin has shown upregulated levels of IL-36 which may be a new target for therapeutics [25, 28].

S100 proteins have antimicrobial activity against gram negative bacteria and regulate proliferation, migration, and differentiation of cells. They may contribute to autoinflammatory signaling in HS by hyperactivation of innate immunity. IL-1 receptor associated kinases are involved in innate immunity and play a role in inflammation [28].

Several new biologic medications targeting IL-17, IL-23, and IL-36 are undergoing clinical trials but there is a need for greater phase 2 studies to elucidate safety and dosing information, as increased dosing is often needed for HS [28] (Fig. 9).

Drug	Screening labs	Monitoring labs and interval	Adverse Events	Pregnancy/Breastfeeding Considerations*^
TNF inhibitors				
Adalimumab Infliximab Etanercept Golimumab	TB, HBV, HCV, HIV CBC Hepatic and renal function	Annual TB screening Consider annual hepatitis serologies and HIV screening for high risk populations Routine CBC, hepatic, and renal function monitoring Avoid live vaccines	*All TNF inhibitors:* Infections (e.g. upper respiratory infections, TB, rarely opportunistic infections). Cytopenias (primarily neutropenia). Infusion or injection site reactions. Caution should be exercised in patients with current or recent history of malilgnancy. *Infliximab*: Autoimmune hepatitis/liver failure, lupus-like syndrome, serum sickness-like reaction (associated with anti-infliximab antibodies). *Etanercept:* Hypoglycemia	TNF inhibitors are likely safe early in pregnancy. Trans-placental transfer has been reported, and low levels of TNF-inhibitors have been detected in neonates exposed during gestation. TNF-inhibitors have also been detected at low-levels in breast milk. While the clinical significance of these findings is unclear, we recommend discussing discontinuation of TNF-inhibitors by the late second or early third trimester, as well as discussing the potential risks of live immunizations in exposed neonates. In some instances the benefit of continuing therapy throughout pregnancy outweighs the risks.

Fig. 9 Summary of recommendations for biologic medications in HS. Adapted from North American clinical management guidelines for hidradenitis suppurativa: A publication from the United States and Canadian Hidradenitis Suppurativa Foundations: Part II: Topical, intralesional, and systemic medical management [5]

IL-1 inhibitor				
Anakinra	TB, HBV, HCV, HIV CBC Hepatic and renal function	Annual TB screening Consider annual hepatitis serologies and HIV screening for high risk populations Routine CBC, hepatic, and renal function monitoring Avoid live vaccines	Injection site reactions (>70%) Skin and respiratory infections	Trans-placental transfer detected Detected in breast milk No preterm births, serious pregnancy complications, or adverse newborn outcomes observed
IL-12-23 inhibitor				
Ustekinumab	TB, HBV, HCV, HIV CBC Hepatic and renal function	Annual TB screening Consider annual hepatitis serologies and HIV screening for high risk populations Routine CBC, hepatic, and renal function monitoring Avoid live vaccines	Nasopharyngeal and upper respiratory infections Nonmelanoma skin cancer	Trans-placental transfer detected Not human data pertaining to lactation No increased risk of congenital defects. Or miscarriages detected in case reports
Abbreviations: TB-tuberculosis, HBV- hepatitis B virus, HCV- Hepatitis C Virus, CBC- complete blood count *Limited data available for safety of all biologic agents in pregnancy or during breastfeeding. ^Discuss potential risks of live immunizations in exposed neonates				

Fig. 9 (continued)

11 Pyoderma Gangrenosum

Pyoderma gangrenosum is a reactive non-infectious inflammatory neutrophilic dermatosis characterized by recurrent skin ulcers. Classically it presents as a painful erythematous lesions precipitated by pathergy (Fig. 10). There are associated syndromes of PG with cystic acne and hidradenitis suppurativa (PASH), PG with pyogenic arthritis and acne (PAPA), and PG with pyogenic arthritis, acne, and hidradenitis suppurativa (PAPASH) [29]. It often affects patients with an underlying inflammatory disorder such as inflammatory bowel disease or rheumatoid arthritis [30].

11.1 Pathophysiology

Much is yet to be discovered about the pathogenesis of PG, however neutrophils are a key regulator of the inflammatory process. Several different inflammatory chemokines and interleukins such as IL-1beta, IL-17, TNF-alpha, IL-8, IL-6, IL-17, and IL 23 have been found in lesional skin [29]. There may be a genetic component with mutations in the PSTP1P1/CDD2BPP1 gene implicated in PAPA and PASH syndromes [29].

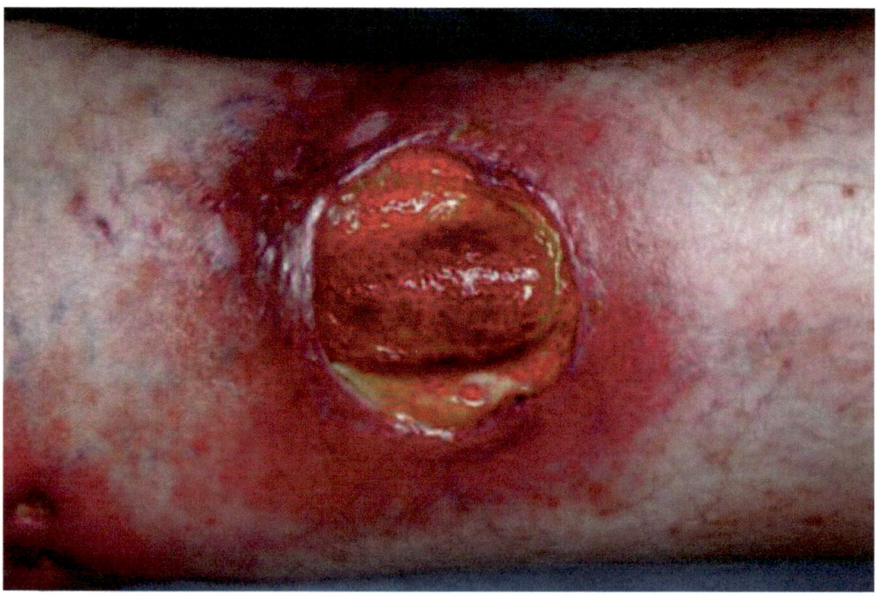

Fig. 10 Painful ulcer in PG. Adapted from Pyoderma gangrenosuma guide to diagnosis and management [29]

11.2 Treatment

Rest is first line treatment for PG. In terms of immunosuppressive medications, cyclosporine is recommended with an A grade due to its similar outcomes of corticosteroids. Other immunosuppressants are graded C1-C2 with limited evidence coming from cases reports [30]. If there is limited response from corticosteroids or cyclosporine, introduction of a biologic is recommended. Adalimumab has been tested in trials and is recommended for suitable patients who have not been response to oral corticosteroids or immunosuppressants. Infliximab was tested in an open-label study and revealed that 69% of patients showed clinical improvement after 6 weeks [29]. Etanercept has also been tested with some results of clinical improvement in patients. Certolizumab pegol has been tested in case reports.

There are reports of response to other biologic medications targeting ILL-12/23, IL-23, IL-1 and IL-17 in case reports however patients typically had inflammatory bowel disease and/or rheumatoid arthritis. Further studies are needed on the use of biologics in the treatment of PG.

Further investigation into the use of JAK inhibitors and other small molecules are needed as it is currently recommended with C1 evidence. There are some reports on successful treatment with tofacitinib and baricitinib. Apremilast (PDE 4 inhibitor) and alefacept (lymphocyte function associated antigen 3 inhibitor) have been described in case reports as well. Larger scale clinical trial data is needed.

12 Special Populations

12.1 Pediatric

PG is a rare disease in childhood, accounting for 4–5% of total cases [31]. Children are likely to have an underlying disease such as Crohn's disease or ulcerative colitis when presenting with PG. Treatment is usually with systemic oral corticosteroids with transition to a steroid-sparing agent such as a calcineurin inhibitor [30, 31].

12.2 Pregnancy

The body in pregnancy is more susceptible to the development of PG due to the neutrophilia and elevated G-CSF and Th17 associated with the end pregnancy. It has been reported that a case of PG was induced after cesarean section [30]. Treatment of PG in pregnancy requires interdisciplinary management and may range from methylprednisolone which has minimal placental transfer [32]. Treatment with cyclosporine or TNF-alpha inhibitors may also be considered however there is a lack of long term safety data [32].

13 Cutaneous Vasculitis

Cutaneous vasculitis may represent a manifestation of systemic vasculitis to those limited to the skin. Therapy is guided by organ involvement, as systemic vasculitis requiring treatment will also treat the cutaneous manifestation. There are limited clinical trial data and guidance is based on case studies and expert consensus (Fig. 11).

13.1 Small Vessel Vasculitis

Cutaneous IgM/IgG immune complex vasculitis is limited to the skin and presents with palpable purpura. Once systemic vasculitis is ruled out, most cases will self resolve in 3–4 weeks. Chronic relapsing cases may be treated with systemic glucocorticoids (0.5–1 mg/kg/day) then tapered to a steroid sparing agent. First line treatment includes colchicine (0.6 mg BID), Dapsone (100–150 mg/day), and azathioprine (2 mg/kg/day) [30]. Immunomodulators and biologics such as methotrexate, mycophenolate, rituximab, infliximab may be used in patients who fail to respond to first or second line treatment.

IgA vasculitis is often self-limited however treatment may include colchicine, dapsone, or azathioprine for chronic cases. Administration of systemic glucocorticoids to prevent renal complications has not been shown to be beneficial [33].

13.2 Medium Sized Vessel Vasculitis

Cutaneous polyarteritis nodosa (PAN) presents most commonly as fixed livedo racemosa and tender subcutaneous nodules on the lower legs. Treatment is guided by severity of disease. Conservative management with rest, NSAIDs may be trialed along with colchicine or dapsone for patients with subcutaneous nodules. For flares, 30 mg prednisone may be escalated to 1 mg/kg/day for more severe disease followed by a taper. Immunosuppression with azathioprine (2 mg/kg) or methotrexate (15-25 mg/week) may be used for severe disease [33]. TNF-alpha inhibition, cyclophosphamide, or IVIG may be considered for relapsing cases [33].

Cryglobulinemic vasculitis presents as tender palpable purpura on the lower legs or retiform purpura with necrosis. For skin limited vasculitis, patients should be screened for HCV and may find relief with colchicine or dapsone.

Eosinophilic granulomatosis with polyangiitis (EGPA) is a mixed small-medium vessel vasculitis involving several organ systems and presents with asthma, eosinophilia, chronic rhinosinusitis and can progress to mononeuritis multiplex and glomerulonephritis. ANCA positive EGPA may present with petechiae and palpable purpura on the lower legs [34]. Administration of glucocorticoids (daily pulses of

Disorder	First-line treatment	Second-line treatment	Third-line treatment
Cutaneous IgM/IgG Immune Complex Vasculitis (primary cutaneous small vessel vasculitis/cutaneous leukocytoclastic angiitis/hypersensitivity vasculitis)	Eliminate/treat potential triggers Supportive care (rest, elevation) NSAIDs Topical steroids	Colchicine (0.6 mg BID) Dapsone (50–200 mg/day) AZA (2 mg/kg/day) CS (e.g., prednisone up to 40-60 mg/day tapered over 3-4 weeks)	COL + DAP MTX MYC CSA CYC Rituximab Infliximab IVIG
Skin-limited IgA vasculitis (Henoch–Schönlein purpura)	Supportive care NSAIDs Topical steroids	Colchicine Dapsone AZA CS	Rituximab MYC CSA CYC PEX
Urticarial vasculitis	Antihistamines NSAIDs Dapsone (100–200 mg/day) CS	Colchicine (0.6 mg BID–TID) HCQ MYC AZA MTX Dapsone + pentoxifylline	Omalizumab Anakinra/Canakinumab Rituximab CYC CSA IVIG Tocilizumab
Cryoglobulinemic vasculitis (skin-predominate)	Direct acting antivirals (e.g., sofosbuvir-velpatasvir) if HCV+ Supportive care	Colchicine Dapsone	Rituximab CS IVIG PEX
Erythema elevatum diutinum	Dapsone Intralesional CS NSAIDs	Colchicine Chloroquine Tetracyclines± niacinamide	MYC MTX CS
Nodular vasculitis (erythema induratum)	Eliminate/treat potential triggers (anti-TB therapy, if indicated) Supportive care NSAIDs Potassium iodide (300 mg TID)	Colchicine	CS MYC

Fig. 11 Summary of treatment options in cutaneous vasculitis. Adapted from Treatment of cutaneous vasculitis [33]

Cutaneous polyarteritis nodosa	Supportive care NSAIDs Colchicine Dapsone CS (0.5–1 mg/kg/day tapered over months)	AZA (2 mg/kg/day) MTX (15–25 mg/wk)	TNF-α inhibitors MYC CYC HCQ IVIG
Abbreviations: AZA, azathioprine; BID, twice daily; CS, corticosteroids; COL, colchicine; CSA, cyclosporine; CYC, cyclophosphamide; DAP, dapsone; HCQ, hydroxychloroquine; HCV, hepatitis C; Ig, immunoglobulin; IVIG, intravenous immunoglobulin; MTX, methotrexate; MYC, mycophenolate mofetil; NSAIDs, nonsteroidal anti-inflammatory drugs; PEX, plasma exchange; TID, three times a day.			

Fig. 11 (continued)

500–1000 mg methylprednisolone for 3 days) is first line therapy to induce remission. For severe disease, treatment may include targeted therapy with mepolizumab (IL-5 inhibitor) for maintenance or in combination with glucocorticoids [34].

13.3 Other Vasculitides

For urticarial vasculitis, antihistamines may be beneficial for skin lesions. Further treatment may include dapsone, hydroxychloroquine, colchicine, or mycophenolate mofetil depending on the case. For refractory cases, treatment with omalizumab, anakinra, canakinumab, and rituximab has been described [33].

Erythema elevatum diutinum (EED) is characterized by red-brown papules and plaques on acral and extensor surfaces. Treatment may include dapsone, NSAIDs, tetracyclines, or colchicine.

13.4 Future Directions

Guidance for the treatment of cutaneous vasculitis remains limited. Clinical trials comparing first line agents such as colchicine, dapsone, and azathioprine have recently been conducted. There are reports of avacopan and IL-5 inhibition for the treatment of ANCA-associated vasculitis [33]. Guidelines for the treatment of eosinophilic granulomatosis with polyangiitis (EGPA) include targeted therapy with mepolizumab (IL-5 inhibitor) for maintenance or in combination with glucocorticoids for remission induction [34]. Further information is needed to identify biomarkers of interest that may be able to be targeted for disease management.

References

1. Lyons AB, Shabeeb N, Nicholson CL, Braunberger TL, Peacock A, Hamzavi IH. Emerging medical treatments for hidradenitis suppurativa. J Am Acad Dermatol. 2020;83(2):554–62.
2. Wolk K, Join-Lambert O, Sabat R. Aetiology and pathogenesis of hidradenitis suppurativa. Br J Dermatol. 2020;183(6):999–1010.
3. Zouboulis CC, Desai N, Emtestam L, Hunger RE, Ioannides D, Juhász I, et al. European S1 guideline for the treatment of hidradenitis suppurativa/acne inversa. J Eur Acad Dermatol Venereol. 2015;29(4):619–44.
4. Moran B, Sweeney CM, Hughes R, Malara A, Kirthi S, Tobin AM, et al. Hidradenitis suppurativa is characterized by dysregulation of the Th17: treg cell axis, which is corrected by anti-TNF therapy. J Invest Dermatol. 2017;137(11):2389–95.
5. Alikhan A, Sayed C, Alavi A, Alhusayen R, Brassard A, Burkhart C, et al. North American clinical management guidelines for hidradenitis suppurativa: a publication from the United States and Canadian Hidradenitis Suppurativa Foundations: Part II: topical, intralesional, and systemic medical management. J Am Acad Dermatol. 2019;81(1):91–101.
6. Malvaso D, Calabrese L, Chiricozzi A, Antonelli F, Coscarella G, Rubegni P, Peris K. IL-17 Inhibition: a valid therapeutic strategy in the management of hidradenitis suppurativa. Pharmaceutics. 2023;15(10).
7. Markota Čagalj A, Marinović B, Bukvić Mokos Z. New and emerging targeted therapies for hidradenitis suppurativa. Int J Mol Sci. 2022;23(7).
8. Martora F, Scalvenzi M, Ruggiero A, Potestio L, Battista T, Megna M. Hidradenitis suppurativa and JAK inhibitors: A review of the published literature. Medicina (Kaunas). 2023;59(4).
9. Tsai YC, Hung CY, Tsai TF. Efficacy and safety of biologics and small molecules for moderate-to-severe hidradenitis suppurativa: a systematic review and network meta-analysis. Pharmaceutics. 2023;15(5).
10. Frew JW, Navrazhina K, Grand D, Sullivan-Whalen M, Gilleaudeau P, Garcet S, et al. The effect of subcutaneous brodalumab on clinical disease activity in hidradenitis suppurativa: an open-label cohort study. J Am Acad Dermatol. 2020;83(5):1341–8.
11. Glatt S, Jemec GBE, Forman S, Sayed C, Schmieder G, Weisman J, et al. Efficacy and safety of bimekizumab in moderate to severe hidradenitis suppurativa: a Phase 2, double-blind, placebo-controlled randomized clinical trial. JAMA Dermatol. 2021;157(11):1279–88.
12. Huang CH, Huang IH, Tai CC, Chi CC. Biologics and small molecule inhibitors for treating hidradenitis suppurativa: a systematic review and meta-analysis. Biomedicines. 2022;10(6).
13. Ring HC, Maul JT, Yao Y, Wu JJ, Thyssen JP, Thomsen SF, Egeberg A. Drug survival of biologics in patients with hidradenitis suppurativa. JAMA Dermatol. 2022;158(2):184–88.
14. Vossen A, Ardon CB, van der Zee HH, Lubberts E, Prens EP. The anti-inflammatory potency of biologics targeting tumour necrosis factor-α, interleukin (IL)-17A, IL-12/23 and CD20 in hidradenitis suppurativa: an ex vivo study. Br J Dermatol. 2019;181(2):314–23.
15. Ben Abdallah H, Bregnhøj A, Emmanuel T, Ghatnekar G, Johansen C, Iversen L. Efficacy and safety of the heat shock protein 90 inhibitor RGRN-305 in hidradenitis suppurativa: a parallel-design double-blind trial. JAMA Dermatol. 2024;160(1):63–70.
16. Kimball AB, Peeva E, Forman S, Moiin A, Khattri S, Porter ML, et al. Brepocitinib, zimlovisertib, and ropsacitinib in hidradenitis suppurativa. NEJM Evid. 2024;3(3):EVIDoa2300155.
17. George A, Lansang RP, Lansang P, Gooderham M. A practical guide to using biologics in pediatric dermatology. J Cutan Med Surg. 2024;28(1):59–67.
18. Fragoso NM, Masson R, Gillenwater TJ, Shi VY, Hsiao JL. Emerging treatments and the clinical trial landscape for hidradenitis suppurativa Part I: topical and systemic medical therapies. Dermatol Ther (Heidelb). 2023;13(8):1661–97.
19. Collier EK, Price KN, Grogan T, Fernandez JM, Seivright JR, Alhusayen R, et al. Provider perspectives on the management of hidradenitis suppurativa in pregnancy—a survey study. Int J Womens Dermatol. 2021;7(3):346–8.
20. Schneeweiss MC et al. Prevalence of pretreatment testing recommended for patients with chronic inflammatory skin diseases. JAMA Dermatol. 2024;160(3):334–40.

21. Emer JJ, Frankel A, Zeichner JA. A practical approach to monitoring patients on biological agents for the treatment of psoriasis. J Clin Aesthet Dermatol. 2010;3(8):20–6.
22. American College of Rheumatology. Anakinra (Kineret) ACR/ARP Medication Guide. https://rheumatology.org/api/asset/blt31768b366f1f4d70. Accessed May 9, 2024.
23. Samuel C, Cornman H, Kambala A, Kwatra SG. A review on the safety of using JAK inhibitors in dermatology: clinical and laboratory monitoring. Dermatol Ther (Heidelb). 2023;13(3):729–49.
24. Swedish Orphan Biovitrum AB. Kineret (anakinra) [package insert]. U.S. Food and Drug Administration website. https://www.accessdata.fda.gov/drugsatfda_docs/label/2016/125319s084lbl.pdf. Revised 2012. Accessed May 9, 2024.
25. Aarts P, Dudink K, Vossen A, van Straalen KR, Ardon CB, Prens EP, van der Zee HH. Clinical implementation of biologics and small molecules in the treatment of hidradenitis suppurativa. Drugs. 2021;81(12):1397–410.
26. Bechara FG, Podda M, Prens EP, Horváth B, Giamarellos-Bourboulis EJ, Alavi A, et al. Efficacy and safety of adalimumab in conjunction with surgery in moderate to severe hidradenitis suppurativa: the SHARPS randomized clinical trial. JAMA Surg. 2021;156(11):1001–9.
27. Maghfour J, Dzuali F, Ezekwe N, Gordon J, Hamzavi IH. Evaluating the efficacy of continuous wave carbon dioxide laser therapy in conjunction with biologics for the management of hidradenitis suppurativa. Br J Dermatol. 2023;189(6):764–83.
28. Zouboulis CC, Frew JW, Giamarellos-Bourboulis EJ, Jemec GBE, Del Marmol V, Marzano AV, et al. Target molecules for future hidradenitis suppurativa treatment. Exp Dermatol. 2021;30(Suppl 1):8–17.
29. George C, Deroide F, Rustin M. Pyoderma gangrenosum—a guide to diagnosis and management. Clin Med (Lond). 2019;19(3):224–8.
30. Yamamoto T, Yamasaki K, Yamanaka K, Komine M, Kawakami T, Yamamoto O, et al. Clinical guidance of pyoderma gangrenosum 2022. J Dermatol. 2023;50(9):e253–75.
31. Schoch JJ, Tolkachjov SN, Cappel JA, Gibson LE, Davis DM. Pediatric pyoderma gangrenosum: a retrospective review of clinical features, etiologic associations, and treatment. Pediatr Dermatol. 2017;34(1):39–45.
32. Vigl K, Posch C, Richter L, Monshi B, Rappersberger K. Pyoderma gangrenosum during pregnancy—treatment options revisited. J Eur Acad Dermatol Venereol. 2016;30(11):1981–4.
33. Micheletti RG. Treatment of cutaneous vasculitis. Front Med (Lausanne). 2022;9:1059612.
34. Emmi G, Bettiol A, Gelain E, Bajema IM, Berti A, Burns S, et al. Evidence-based guideline for the diagnosis and management of eosinophilic granulomatosis with polyangiitis. Nat Rev Rheumatol. 2023;19(6):378–93.

Immunomodulators for Common Dermatologic Disorders: A Focus on Acne, Rosacea, Seborrheic Dermatitis

Niel N. Veirup, Amit Sharma, and Brad P. Glick

Abstract This chapter explores the immunomodulatory aspects of acne, rosacea, and seborrheic dermatitis, emphasizing their multifactorial etiology and the role of inflammation in disease progression. Treatment approaches for these conditions involve targeting various contributing factors, with a focus on combination therapies tailored to disease severity. Recent advancements in microencapsulated formulations and novel agents offer promising avenues for enhancing treatment efficacy and tolerability. Insights from gene expression studies highlight immune pathways implicated in these disorders, providing valuable targets for future therapeutic interventions. Overall, understanding immunomodulation in dermatological conditions is crucial for advancing treatment strategies and improving patient outcomes.

Keywords Immunomodulators · Treatment · Acne · Rosacea · Seborrheic dermatitis

1 Acne

Acne is the most common skin condition worldwide and its etiology is multifactorial [1]. The pathogenesis of this condition is characterized by well-defined mechanisms of disease including androgen induction of sebum production, follicular hyperkeratinization, and proliferation of *Cutibacterium acnes* [2]. Additionally, in response to the production of *C. acnes*, there is a concomitant Th17 and Th17/Th1-driven inflammatory response that contributes to the clinical manifestations of acne [3]. There is a wide range of clinical findings and levels of severity from small open and closed comedones isolated on the face to large nodulocystic lesions that can cover the face, chest, and back.

Immunomodulatory mechanisms of disease are critical to our continued understanding of acne and its variants, as well as play an important role in the development of new and emerging therapeutic targets. Treatment of acne therefore often requires a

N. N. Veirup · A. Sharma · B. P. Glick (✉)
Larkin Health System, Miami, FL, USA
e-mail: spinsking1103@aol.com

N. Bhatia (ed.), *Immunomodulators and Biologics in Dermatologic Treatment*,
https://doi.org/10.1007/978-3-031-66590-5_11

multifaceted approach depending on disease severity, in order to address the different contributing factors leading to the development of acneiform lesions. Standard of care has often relied on retinoids (vitamin A derivatives), benzoyl peroxide, and both topical and oral antibiotics [4]. Retinoids modulate and aid in increasing the rate of cell turnover addressing issues with follicular hyperkeratinization. Topical formulations include adapalene, tretinoin, tazarotene, and more recently, trifarotene. In moderate to severe and refractory cases oral isotretinoin is also often utilized with largely successful results. Although often quite effective, retinoids often irritate the skin causing redness, dryness, and scaling which can limit their tolerability. Benzoyl peroxide is an effective adjuvant therapy when combined with both topical retinoids and topical antibiotics but can also be irritating. New formulations have combined the above ingredients in an attempt to simplify the patient experience and increase user compliance. For example, tretinoin (T) 0.1% with 3% benzoyl peroxide (BPO) utilizes microencapsulation technology that allows for both active ingredients to be stable within the same formula while also providing increased tolerability for the patient [5]. In two studies, a combination of BPO/T was significantly more effective than vehicle in treating acne with a higher percentage of participants achieving success in terms of Investigator Global Assessment (IGA) scores when using BPO/T compared to those using the vehicle [5]. In the first study, 38.5% of participants using BPO/T achieved success compared to 11.5% of those using the vehicle (p < 0.001), and in the second study, 25.4% of participants using BPO/T achieved success compared to 14.7% of those using the vehicle ($p = 0.017$) [5]. Additionally, a formulation of clindamycin phosphate 1.2%, adapalene 0.15% and benzoyl peroxide 3.1% topical gel (IDP-126) was formulated utilizing a polymeric mesh technology for both stability and even distribution of active ingredients [6]. At the end of a 12-week treatment period, a significantly higher proportion of participants (52.5%) achieved treatment success defined as participants achieving a $\geq$ 2-grade reduction from baseline in Evaluator's Global Severity Score and clear/almost clear skin) and least-squares mean absolute changes from baseline in inflammatory and noninflammatory lesion counts at week 12 with IDP-126 compared to those using a control substance (8.1%) or other combinations of treatments (e.g. BPO/adapalene, clindamycin/BPO; or clindamycin phosphate/adapalene) (range 27.8–30.5%; p $\leq$ 0.001, all) [6].

Oral antibiotics, particularly tetracyclines (doxycycline, minocycline, and most recently, sarecycline), have been employed in the treatment of acne, especially when inflammatory lesions are present. The mechanism of action for tetracyclines is twofold. First, their antimicrobial properties act by binding the 16S ribosomal RNA of the bacterial ribosome 30S subunit to inhibit protein synthesis and therefore decrease the burden of *C. acnes* in the skin [7]. Additionally, tetracyclines exhibit an anti-inflammatory effect by decreasing neutrophil chemotaxis and matrix metalloproteinases while also downregulating inflammatory cytokines. One study investigating the immunomodulatory role of doxycycline showed the inhibition trypsin-like serine proteases (TLSP) action via assay of cathelicidin enzymatic processing by keratinocytes [8]. By utilizing recombinant hCAP18 protein, the study revealed that doxycycline could decrease the proteolytic processing of hCAP18 to

LL-37 [8]. They concluded that doxycycline functioned indirectly by preventing tryptic kallikrein-related peptidases (KLK) activation by MMPs [8].

Addressing the hormonal component of acne has been limited to medications such as spironolactone and oral contraceptives with their use being restricted to females and also having risk of systemic side effects. The etiology of acne has shown that likely all individuals with the condition have some hormonal component contributing to their condition. Most recently topical clascoterone (1% cream) was approved for the treatment of acne vulgaris in patients age 12 or greater, regardless of gender. This is the first FDA-approved topical medication that targets the hormonal induction of sebum production. Clascoterone acts in the skin to competitively inhibit androgen binding modulating the production of sebum leading to its downstream effects and improvement of acne. Additionally, according to in vitro and clinical studies, the main possible primary metabolite of clascoterone is cortexolone, which is an inactive metabolite. The plasma concentrations of cortexolone were generally below or near the lower limit of quantitation (0.5 ng/mL). Although clascoterone penetrates the skin, the systemic activity of the drug is limited due to rapid hydrolysis of clascoterone into the inactive metabolite by skin and plasma esterases, namely carboxylesterase. Clascoterone binding leads to reduced transcription of androgen-responsive genes thus decreasing sebum production and activation of inflammatory pathways, which includes proinflammatory cytokine synthesis specifically IL-8, IL-16, and IL-1B [9].

Acne presents a multifaceted challenge with its etiology rooted in various factors including androgen induction of sebum production, follicular hyperkeratinization, and the proliferation of *C. acnes*, all of which trigger an inflammatory response. The complexity of this condition underscores the importance of immunomodulatory approaches in both understanding its pathogenesis and developing effective treatments. Current therapies often encompass a combination of retinoids, benzoyl peroxide, and antibiotics, which target different aspects of the disease process. However, their efficacy can be limited by side effects and tolerability issues. Recent advancements, such as topical clascoterone, offer promising alternatives by specifically targeting hormonal induction of sebum production, representing a significant step forward in acne treatment. Moving forward, continued research into immunomodulatory mechanisms and the development of targeted therapies hold the potential to significantly improve outcomes for individuals affected by acne.

2 Rosacea

Rosacea is also a common skin condition that exists on a spectrum from central erythema and telangiectasias on the face to also including papulopustules. Advanced disease can present with phymatous changes and extracutaneous manifestations can include ocular involvement. The etiology of rosacea has yet to be fully elucidated but it is believed to be multifactorial in nature with aggravating factors including environmental triggers (e.g., UV radiation, diet, temperature). In addition to environmental factors, immune dysregulation influence by increased cathelicidin (e.g.,

LL-37, a peptide) and kallikrein 5 (KLK5), an enzyme, in the skin of rosacea patients appears to play an important role in disease pathogenesis [10]. Increased expression of toll-like receptor 2 (TLR2) on keratinocytes in affected skin exacerbates LL-37 levels, leading to heightened inflammation and vascular alterations [11, 12]. Moreover, the upregulation of matrix metalloproteinases (MMPs) further complicates the condition by promoting the breakdown of connective tissue proteins, contributing to the pathogenesis of rosacea [13].

Depending on the clinical type of rosacea will determine which treatment options are best suited for a patient. Predominantly telangiectatic and erythematous rosacea without papulopustules can be treated with topical alpha-agonist such as oxymetazoline which acts by temporarily constricting the superficial blood vessels alleviating the appearance of redness. For the papulopustular subset of rosacea, other topical treatments can be utilized such as ivermectin, metronidazole, and azelaic acid. Topical ivermectin works both as an antiparasitic agent targeting the Demodex mite and also has anti-inflammatory properties. In a 12-week week study using ivermectin topical cream 1%, there was a significant reduction in inflammatory markers (LL-37, HBD3 and TNF-α) for TLR4 ($p < 0.05$) in addition to a significant reduction in the mean density of mites ($p < 0.001$) [14].

Newer topical treatments in the armamentarium are minocycline 1.5% foam and microencapsulated benzoyl peroxide 5%. Two 12-week, phase 3, randomized double-blind studies showed a significantly greater reduction in the number of inflammatory lesions ($p < 0.0001$) and higher rates of IGA treatment success ($p = 0.0077$) with minocycline foam 1.5% [15]. Encapsulated benzoyl peroxide 5% (E-BPO 5%) uses a novel microencapsulation technology to entrap (BPO) in silica microcapsules to prolong drug delivery time and improve therapeutic response along with reducing skin irritation. In two 12-week, randomized, double-blind, vehicle cream-controlled Phase III trials E-BPO 5% showed a significant IGA success ($p < 0.001$) and reduction in the number of inflammatory lesions ($p < 0.001$) compared to placebo [16].

Tetracycline antibiotics are used to treat inflammatory lesions of rosacea. Its mechanism of action and anti-inflammatory properties are described above in the acne section. There has been a focus on subantimicrobial dose doxycycline. Sarecycline has been shown to have a narrow spectrum of antibiotic activity. Low-dose minocycline has shown safety and efficacy. Isotretinoin can be used for severe and recalcitrant disease; it reduces the size of sebaceous glands and sebum production. It significantly reduces facial cutaneous blood flow. It exerts its anti-inflammatory properties by significantly decreasing monocyte TLR-2 expression on keratinocytes [17].

There are other treatment options for vascular lesions. Beta-blockers can help with erythema and flushing. Propranolol and nadolol are conventional β-1 and β-2 blockers that reduce flushing. Carvedilol is a β-1, β-2, and weak α -1 blocker used to reduce facial flushing and erythema or rosacea [18]. A systematic review has looked at botulinum toxin for the reduction of erythema. There was some temporary paralysis and it seemed to help reduce erythema [19]. It inhibits mast cell degradation, and release of substance P and calcitonin gene-related peptide [19]. A prospective, randomized, placebo-controlled multicenter study looked at the use of omega-3 fatty acids for ocular rosacea. There was a significant change in subjective dry eye symptoms and meibomian gland score, Schirmer score, and tear film breakup time [20]. Patients with rosacea have been found to have a higher prevalence of small intestinal bacterial overgrowth (SIBO). In patients with rosacea and SIBO, treatment with rifaximin improved rosacea [21].

Rosacea presents on a spectrum of manifestations ranging from central erythema to papulopustules, with advanced stages involving phymatous changes and ocular complications. While its etiology remains multifactorial, environmental triggers such as UV radiation and diet play significant roles with newer understanding revealing the influence of inflammation on the disease process. Treatment strategies vary depending on clinical presentation, with topical agents like alpha-agonists and ivermectin addressing different subtypes. Novel topical formulations, including minocycline foam and microencapsulated benzoyl peroxide, have shown efficacy in reducing inflammatory lesions. Additionally, tetracycline antibiotics can be utilized in mild to moderate cases with isotretinoin reserved for severe cases. Beyond traditional therapies, beta-blockers, botulinum toxin, and omega-3 fatty acids offer promising avenues for managing vascular and ocular manifestations. Addressing associated conditions like small intestinal bacterial overgrowth can also contribute to improved outcomes in rosacea management.

3 Seborrheic Dermatitis

Seborrheic dermatitis (SD) is a common inflammatory papulosquamous condition that causes redness, itching, and flaking. It is usually located on sebum-rich areas such as the scalp, face, and upper body. The pathogenesis is not fully understood but it is related to an abnormal immune response to *Malassezia* species, a common commensal yeast on the skin [22]. Seborrheic dermatitis tends to be chronic with remissions and exacerbations. There is no cure but it can be managed with medicated shampoos, creams, gels, lotions, solutions, oils, and foams. More severe cases can be treated with topical corticosteroids, topical calcineurin inhibitors (TCIs) and antifungal creams.

A recent observational study led by Emma Guttman-Yassky, MD, PhD and Benjamin Ungar, MD has shown distinct gene expression patterns in seborrheic dermatitis. They identified 1374 different genes between seborrheic dermatitis and healthy controls. There was upregulation of Th17 and Th22-related pathways indicating a strong immune response in seborrheic dermatitis. Downregulation of skin barrier markers such as CLDN1/8, FA2H and ELOVL3 is involved in tight junctions and lipid metabolism pathways. There was a significant correlation between the severity of seborrheic dermatitis and immunologic markers of disease.

The aim of treatment in seborrheic dermatitis is to modulate sebum production, reducing *Malassezia* colonization and controlling inflammation. Shampoos can be used as monotherapy or in conjunction with topical corticosteroids. Over-the-counter formulations usually contain salicylic acid, selenium sulfide, tar, or pyrithione zinc.

Topical ketoconazole, an antifungal is the mainstay of treatment as a shampoo on the scalp and cream on the body. Ketoconazole 2% shampoo has been FDA-approved since 1990 for moderate-to-severe scalp SD. It blocks fungal ergosterol synthesis via inhibition of lanosterol C-14-demethylase [23]. In addition, ketoconazole has anti-inflammatory properties by inhibiting leukotrienes. Ciclopirox is a synthetic, hydroxypyridone-derivative with broad antifungal activity. It is FDA-approved as 0.77% gel and 1% shampoo with stronger concentrations available in other countries. Its mechanism of action involves the inhibition of fungal metal-dependent enzymes that damage mitochondria and cell membranes [23]. It also has anti-inflammatory properties by inhibiting prostaglandin and leukotriene release. Short courses of low-potency topical corticosteroids can be used to suppress inflammation. Tacrolimus and pimecrolimus are TCIs used 'off label' for maintenance therapy in SD. They are non-steroidal agents that suppress the synthesis of pro-inflammatory cytokines by binding to intracellular FK506-binding protein [24]. Roflumilast 0.3% foam is a novel once-a-day FDA-approved for patients 9 years and older. It is a phosphodiesterase-4 (PDE-4) inhibitor that exerts its anti-inflammatory effects by increasing cyclic adenosine monophosphate (cAMP) levels [25] thus reducing inflammatory cytokines. Significantly more patients in the roflumilast group achieved treatment success of 80% vs. 59% for vehicle at week 8 ($p < 0.0001$). Clearance at week 8 was 51% for roflumilast vs. 28% for vehicle. Erythema score of zero was 58% (roflumilast) vs. 33% (vehicle) group and 58% in the roflumilast group achieved a scaling score of zero compared to 38% (vehicle) [26].

In severe and/or resistant cases systemic antifungals or UVB phototherapy can be considered. Terbinafine is a lipophilic antifungal allylamine with antimycotic properties. It blocks the biosynthesis of ergosterol by inhibiting squalene epoxidase. Itraconazole is a highly keratinophilic and lipophilic triazole that works by inhibiting 14 alpha-demethylase which blocks lanosterol conversion to ergosterol. Its anti-inflammatory effects are related to the inhibition of metabolites of 5-lipoxygenase.

In summary, SD is characterized by redness, itching, and flaking, mainly affecting sebum-rich areas such as the scalp, face, and upper body. While the exact cause remains unknown, it is associated with an abnormal immune response to the yeast *Malassezia* species. Treatment aims to modulate sebum production, reduce *Malassezia* colonization, and control inflammation. Various options including medicated shampoos, creams, gels, lotions, and foams are available, with topical ketoconazole and other antifungals being a mainstay due to their antifungal and anti-inflammatory properties. Topical corticosteroids, calcineurin inhibitors, and newer agents like roflumilast 0.3% foam may also be used. In severe or resistant cases, systemic antifungals or UVB phototherapy can be considered. Recent research by Waldman has identified distinct gene expression patterns in SD, revealing upregulation of immune pathways and downregulation of skin barrier markers. These findings provide valuable insights into the pathogenesis of SD and potential targets for future therapeutic interventions. Effective management of SD requires a multifaceted approach tailored to individual patient needs, aiming to alleviate symptoms, reduce inflammation, and restore skin barrier function.

References

1. Bhate K, Williams HC. Epidemiology of acne vulgaris. Br J Dermatol. 2013;168(3):474–85. https://doi.org/10.1111/bjd.12149. PMID: 23210645.
2. Layton AM, Eady EA, Whitehouse H, Del Rosso JQ, Fedorowicz Z, van Zuuren EJ. Oral spironolactone for acne vulgaris in adult females: a hybrid systematic review. Am J Clin Dermatol. 2017;18(2):169–91.
3. Kistowska M, Meier B, Proust T, et al. Propionibacterium acnes promotes Th17 and Th17/Th1 responses in acne patients. J Invest Dermatol. 2015;135(1):110–8.
4. Reynolds RV, Yeung H, Cheng CE, Cook-Bolden F, Desai SR, Druby KM, Freeman EE, Keri JE, Stein Gold LF, Tan JKL, Tollefson MM, Weiss JS, Wu PA, Zaenglein AL, Han JM, Barbieri JS. Guidelines of care for the management of acne vulgaris. J Am Acad Dermatol. 2024;S0190-9622(23). https://doi.org/10.1016/j.jaad.2023.12.017. Epub ahead of print. PMID: 38300170.
5. Del Rosso J, Sugarman J, Green L, Lain T, Levy-Hacham O, Mizrahi R, Gold LS. Efficacy and safety of microencapsulated benzoyl peroxide and microencapsulated tretinoin for the treatment of acne vulgaris: Results from two phase 3 double-blind, randomized, vehicle-controlled studies. J Am Acad Dermatol. 2023;89(4):719–27. https://doi.org/10.1016/j.jaad.2023.05.093. Epub 2023 Jun 24 PMID: 37356627.
6. Gold LS, Baldwin H, Kircik LH, Weiss JS, Pariser DM, Callender V, Lain E, Gold M, Beer K, Draelos Z, Sadick N, Pillai R, Bhatt V, Tanghetti EA. Efficacy and safety of a fixed-dose clindamycin phosphate 1.2%, benzoyl peroxide 3.1%, and adapalene 0.15% gel for moderate-to-severe acne: a randomized Phase II study of the first triple-combination drug. Am J Clin Dermatol. 2022;23(1):93–104. https://doi.org/10.1007/s40257-021-00650-3. Epub 2021 Oct 21. PMID: 34674160; PMCID: PMC8776677.
7. Perret LJ, Tait CP. Tetracyclines in dermatology. Austr J Dermatol. 2014;55:111–8. https://doi.org/10.1111/ajd.12075.
8. Kanada KN, Nakatsuji T, Gallo RL. Doxycycline indirectly inhibits proteolytic activation of tryptic kallikrein-related peptidases and activation of cathelicidin. J Invest Dermatol. 2012;132(5):1435–42. https://doi.org/10.1038/jid.2012.14. Epub 2012 Feb 16. PMID: 22336948; PMCID: PMC4169281
9. Rosette C, Agan FJ, Mazzetti A, Moro L, Gerloni M. Cortexolone 17α-propionate (clascoterone) is a novel androgen receptor antagonist that inhibits production of lipids and inflammatory cytokines from sebocytes in vitro. J Drugs Dermatol. 2019;18(5):412–8 PMID: 31141847.
10. Yamasaki K, Di Nardo A, Bardan A, Murakami M, Ohtake T, Coda A, Dorschner RA, Bonnart C, Descargues P, Hovnanian A, Morhenn VB, Gallo RL. Increased serine protease activity and cathelicidin promotes skin inflammation in rosacea. Nat Med. 2007(8):975–80. https://doi.org/10.1038/nm1616. Epub 2007 Aug 5 PMID: 17676051.
11. Ahn CS, Huang WW. Rosacea pathogenesis. Dermatol Clin. 2018;36(2):81–6. https://doi.org/10.1016/j.det.2017.11.001. Epub 2017 Dec 15 PMID: 29499802.
12. Yamasaki K, Gallo RL. Rosacea as a disease of cathelicidins and skin innate immunity. J Investig Dermatol Symp Proc. 2011;15(1):12–5. https://doi.org/10.1038/jidsymp.2011.4. PMID: 22076322.
13. Del Rosso JQ, Thiboutot D, Gallo R, Webster G, Tanghetti E, Eichenfield LF, Stein-Gold L, Berson D, Zaenglein A. Consensus recommendations from the American Acne & Rosacea Society on the management of rosacea, part 3: a status report on systemic therapies. Cutis. 2014;93(1):18–28 PMID: 24505581.
14. Schaller M, Gonser L, Belge K, Braunsdorf C, Nordin R, Scheu A, Borelli C. Dual anti-inflammatory and anti-parasitic action of topical ivermectin 1% in papulopustular rosacea. J Eur Acad Dermatol Venereol. 2017;31(11):1907–11. https://doi.org/10.1111/jdv.14437. Epub 2017 Aug 29 PMID: 28653460.
15. Gold LS, Del Rosso JQ, Kircik L, et al. Minocycline 1.5% foam for the topical treatment of moderate to severe papulopustular rosacea: results of two phase 3, randomized, clinical trials.

J Am Acad Dermatol. 2020;82:1166–73. https://doi.org/10.1016/j.jaad.2020.01.043. PMID: 32004648.
16. Bhatia ND, Werschler WP, Baldwin H, et al. Efficacy and safety of microencapsulated benzoyl peroxide cream, 5%, in Rosacea: results from two Phase III, randomized, vehicle-controlled trials. J Clin Aesthet Dermatol. 2023;16(8):34–40 PMID: 37636253.
17. Dispenza MC, Wolpert EB, Gilliland KL, Dai JP, Cong Z, Nelson AM, Thiboutot DM. Systemic isotretinoin therapy normalizes exaggerated TLR-2-mediated innate immune responses in acne patients. J Invest Dermatol. 2012;132(9):2198–205. https://doi.org/10.1038/jid.2012.111. Epub 2012 Apr 19. PMID: 22513780; PMCID: PMC3614089.
18. Seo BH, Kim DH, Suh HS, et al. Facial flushing and erythema of rosacea improved by carvedilol. Derm Ther. 2020;33(6):e14520. https://doi.org/10.1111/dth.14520. PMID: 33174351.
19. Zhang H, Tang K, Wang Y, et al. Use of botulinum toxin in treating rosacea: a systematic review. Clin Cosmet Investig Derm. 2021;30(14):407–17. https://doi.org/10.2147/CCID.S307013. PMID: 33958886.
20. Bhargava R, Chandra M, Bansal U, et al. A randomized controlled trial of omega 3 fatty acids in Rosacea patients with dry eye symptos. Curr Eye Res. 2016;41(10):1274–80. https://doi.org/10.3109/02713683.2015.1122810. PMID: 27050028.
21. Weinstock LB, Steinhoff M. Rosacea and small intestinal bacterial overgrowth: prevalence and response to rifaximin. J Am of Dermatol. 2013;68(5):875–6. https://doi.org/10.1016/j.jaad.20212.11.038. PMID: 23602178.
22. Jackson JM, Alexis A, Zirwas M, et al. Unmet needs for patients with seborrheic dermatitis. J Am Acad of Dermatol. 2022;90(3):597–604. https://doi.org/10.1016/j.jaad.2022.12.017.
23. Dall'Oglio F, Nasca MR, Gerbino C, et al. An overview of the diagnosis and management of seborrheic dermatitis. Clin Cosmet Investig Dermatol. 2022;15:1537–48. https://doi.org/10.2147/CCID.S284671. PMID: 35967915.
24. Gutfreund K, Bienias W, Szewczyk A, et al. Topical calcineurin inhibitors in dermatology. Part I: Properties, method, and effectiveness of drug use. Postepy Dermatol Alergol. (2013);30(3):165–169. https://doi.org/10.5114/pdia.2013.35619. PMID: 24278069.
25. Zirwas MJ, Draelos ZD, DuBois J, et al. Efficacy of roflumilast foam, 0.3%, in patients with seborrheic dermatitis. A double-blind, vehicle-controlled Phase 2a randomized clinical trial. JAMA Dermatol. 2023;159(6):613–20. https://doi.org/10.1001/jamadermatol.2023.0846. PMID: 37133856.
26. Blauvelt A, Draelos ZD, Gooderham M, et al. Efficacy and safety of roflumilast foam 0.3% in patients with seborrheic dermatitis in a Phase 3 trial: assessment of pruritus. SKIN J Cutaneous Med. 2023;7(4):s226. https://doi.org/10.25251/skin.7.supp.226

Prescribing and Advocating for Immunomodulators in Dermatology Practice

D. J. Patel, J. Kitsen, N. Bhatia, and G. M. Lewitt

Abstract The integration of biologic and small molecule therapies has revolutionized dermatological care, offering efficacy with a reduced side effect profile. However, accessibility remains a challenge due to a myriad of barriers, including financial constraints, geographic disparities, and insurance barriers. This chapter reviews the multifaceted approach needed to bridge the gap between theory and practice in implementing key therapies. Key strategies include physician education, coordination of care through biologic coordinators and specialty pharmacies, advocacy efforts to challenge restrictive insurance practices, and ongoing research to optimize treatment outcomes. By addressing these challenges collectively, stakeholders can ensure equitable access to life-changing treatments and advance the field of dermatological medicine towards personalized and effective care.

Keywords Access · Advocacy · Biologic · Coordinator · Formulary · Prior Authorization

1 Overview of Small Molecule and Biologics in Dermatologic Treatment

Small molecule and biologic therapies have revolutionized the field of dermatology in recent years, offering novel treatment options for various skin conditions such as psoriasis, atopic dermatitis (AD), and hidradenitis suppurativa [1]. They have provided targeted therapies for conditions in which previous treatment options were limited to topical corticosteroids or broad systemic immunosuppressants. Targeted therapy has rapidly become more commonly used for its improved efficacy and safety profile in comparison to previous treatment options [1].

D. J. Patel · J. Kitsen · N. Bhatia · G. M. Lewitt (✉)
Illinois Dermatology Institute Denova Research, Chicago, USA
e-mail: gmlewitt@illinoisderm.com

N. Bhatia (ed.), *Immunomodulators and Biologics in Dermatologic Treatment*,
https://doi.org/10.1007/978-3-031-66590-5_12

2 Significance and Evolution of These Therapies in Dermatology

The development of small molecule and biologic therapies has been closely intertwined with advances in our understanding of the underlying pathogenesis of dermatologic conditions. By elucidating the molecular mechanisms driving diseases such as psoriasis, atopic dermatitis, and autoimmune blistering disorders, researchers have identified specific targets for therapeutic intervention. This deeper understanding has led to the development of increasingly targeted and effective therapies.

Small molecule and biologic therapies have expanded the treatment landscape beyond traditional dermatologic conditions. Biologics have demonstrated efficacy in diseases previously considered refractory to conventional therapies, including rare autoimmune bullous diseases, eosinophilic skin diseases, and certain forms of cutaneous lymphoma. This has opened new avenues for research and therapeutic innovation in dermatology.

3 Bridge from Theoretical Concepts to Practical Applications

Despite their remarkable efficacy, both small molecule and biologic therapies pose challenges such as high costs, access barriers, and the potential development of tolerance or adverse effects over time [1]. Future research endeavors are concentrated on optimizing treatment regimens, investigating novel therapeutic targets, developing biosimilars to enhance affordability, and widening access to these transformative therapies for all patients in need [2]. This paper aims to shed light on the challenges faced by physicians and patients in accessing these medications and aims to offer guidance on overcoming these obstacles.

4 Types of Biologics and Small Molecules in Dermatology Biologics

Biologic therapies are large, complex molecules usually sourced from living organisms, comprising proteins, antibodies, or nucleic acids, and function within the extracellular space [1]. Currently, they are primarily administered via injection or infusion. Biologics are engineered to target precise components of the immune system or inflammatory pathways, enabling precision therapy. They have transformed the treatment landscape of autoimmune and inflammatory skin diseases by offering highly targeted therapy with reduced systemic side effects.

5 Current Available Medications and Their Efficacy

Commonly used biologics and small molecule drugs in dermatology are listed in Table 1. The efficacy of biologics is dependent on the medication itself, however in a large meta-analysis to compare biologic drugs for moderate-to-severe psoriasis, number needed to treat (NNT) was used to measure efficacy [3]. The study analyzed data from 42 double-blind, randomized, phase 3 clinical trials for biologics including adalimumab, brodalumab, certolizumab pegol, etanercept, guselkumab, infliximab, ixekizumab, risankizumab, secukinumab, tildrakizumab, and ustekinumab [3]. NNT was calculated to achieve Psoriasis Area and Severity Index (PASI) 75/90/100 responses at various time points and Dermatology Life Quality Index (DLQI) response 0, 1 at week 12 [3]. Overall, brodalumab and ixekizumab consistently showed high efficacy in achieving clearance of psoriasis lesions, particularly in the early stages of treatment [3]. After one year, risankizumab demonstrated comparable efficacy to brodalumab and ixekizumab [3]. The study provides valuable insights for clinicians and patients in selecting the most effective treatment for moderate-to-severe psoriasis. This meta-analysis highlights that vast difference of injectable biologic efficacy in comparison to traditional/conventional systemic therapies previously published with much higher NNT metrics.

6 Small Molecules

Small molecule drugs are typically low molecular weight compounds capable of penetrating cell membranes and targeting specific molecules or pathways within cells [1]. Due to their small size, typically < 1 kDa, they exhibit high bioavailability and are commonly administered orally [1]. In dermatology, small molecule therapies are frequently employed for conditions like psoriasis, atopic dermatitis, and alopecia areata. In addition, they are also being investigated in other dermatological/rheumatological conditions such as lupus and dermatomyositis. Examples of small molecule drugs used in dermatology include Janus Kinase (JAK) inhibitors such as abrocitinib and phosphodiesterase 4 (PDE4) inhibitors like apremilast. Refer to Table 1 for an expanded list of medications, FDA indications, and costs.

7 Comparative Analysis with Biologics

Small molecule and biologic therapies each have their own advantages and limitations. Small molecule drugs are often orally administered and may have systemic effects, while biologics are typically administered via injection or infusion and may have lower systemic toxicity. The choice between small molecule and biologic therapy depends on factors such as the severity of the condition, patient preferences,

Table 1 Examples of biologic and small molecule medications and their Wholesale Acquisition Cost (WAC) currently FDA approved in Dermatology [4]

Biologic	FDA-indication (s)	Wholesale acquistion cost (WAC)
etanercept	RA, PsA, PsO, AS, JIA	$1492.04/pack
adalimumab	RA, PsA, PsO, AS ,UC, CD, UV, HS, JIA	$5968.18/ pens
inflixmab	PsA, PsO, CD, UC, RA(+ mtx), AS	$1,168/vial
certolizumab	PsA, PsO, AS, CD, nr-axSpA	$4815.5/2 syringes
ustekinumab	PsO, PsA, CD, UC	45 mg—$12,095.41/90 mg—$24,190.82
secukinumab	PsO, PsA,AS, nr-axSpA, HS	$5929.33/2 pens
ixekizumab	PsO, PsA, AS, nr-axSpA	$5974.40/pen
brodalumab	PsO	$1966.30/syringe
guselkumab	PsO, PsA	$11,938.37/pen or syringe
tildrakizumab	PsO	$16,178.35/syringe
risankizumab-rzaa	PsO, PsA, CD, UC, CD	$17,013.70/syringe or pen
dupilumab	AD, asthma, CRSwNP, PN	$1601.70/syringe or pen
omalizumab	Asthma, CSU, nasal polyps	$1162.34/vial
rituximab	NHL, CLL, RA, GPA, MPA, PV	$990.36/10 Ml/$4913.79/50 mL
tralokinumab	AD	$1674.40/2 syringes
abrocitinib	AD	$4914/month
upadacitinib	RA, PsA, AS, nr-axSpA, UC, CD, AD	$6124.96/month
baricitinib	AA, RA	$2622/month—2 mg, $5244/month—4 mg
apremilast	PsO, PsA, BD	$4600.48/month
ritlecitinib	AA	$3769.23/month

WAC is subject to change on an annual basis

comorbidities, and cost considerations. Dermatologists often tailor treatment plans based on individual patient characteristics and response to therapy. Overall, both small molecule and biologic therapies have significantly expanded the therapeutic options available to dermatologists and have led to improved outcomes for patients with a wide range of skin conditions.

8 Challenges in Clinical Implementation

8.1 *Physician's Constraints in Prescribing*

Within the realm of dermatologic treatment, selecting an appropriate systemic therapy is a complex undertaking for physicians. The intricate decision-making process is influenced by factors such as disease severity, comorbid health conditions, treatment guidelines such as the National Psoriasis Foundation (NPF), step therapy, and the preferences of both patients and healthcare providers [5]. The landscape of immunomodulators and biologics in dermatology has shifted immensely, with a noticeable shift from classically last-resort agents to often first or second line therapy [6]. Unfortunately, the complex constraints, such as the restrictive coverage policies and high out-of-pocket costs, potentially leads to rejection by insurers or abandonment by patients. These constraints highlight the delicate balance physicians must navigate, ensuring optimal patient care while contending with the intricacies of healthcare utilization in dermatological treatment [5, 6].

The prescription patterns associated with biologic medications was revealed by insights from a retrospective cohort study from electronic health records (EHR) data from 34,714 eligible psoriasis patients. From the analysis of the data: up to 50% of patients, upon receiving a prescription for a biologic medication, did not receive a second prescription for the same medication. This finding poses significant implications for physicians, prompting questions about patient adherence, initiation of therapy, and the intricate factors influencing the continuation of prescribed treatments [5].

Effective counseling of patients about the risks, benefits, and alternatives is paramount to ensuring the comprehensive understanding of biologic therapy [6]. Acknowledging the "long and cumbersome" package inserts that dermatologists are far too familiar with, Ortleb and Levitt created a checklist of common considerations that are applicable for most biologics [6].

Screening for tuberculosis is an important consideration due to increased risk of TB reactivation. Patients prescribed infliximab and adalimumab – and less with etanercept – had an increase in TB activation, implying an increased risk for TNF antibodies versus TNF-receptor inhibitors [6]. Screening should occur pre-therapy and annually, especially for TNF-alpha and IL-12/23 inhibitors.

Screening for hepatitis B is not only paramount for patients who are at high risk, but also for all biologics with the exception of IVIG [6]. Additional hepatitis C screening is often performed if baseline ALT and AST are elevated or if other risk factors are identified. Of note, special consideration for infliximab should be made as it has rarely reported hepatotoxicity [6].

Efforts to navigate vaccination protocols, particularly in the context of live or attenuated vaccines, should be made in tandem with initiation or discontinuation of biologics. The integration of these considerations provides guidance for physicians managing infectious disease risks.

The effect of biologics on pregnancy is a consideration that should be reevaluated as more studies are conducted and guidelines are updated.

There is also little data regarding recurrence of previously treated or dormant cancers. Therefore, clinical considerations must be made of biologics, as there may be an association of varying risk of each biologic with various malignancies. Recent studies have reported that overall concern of some biologics such as IL-17 and IL 23, may be less compared to TNF and traditional immunosuppressant medications such as methotrexate and cyclosporin A [7–9]. Non-melanoma skin cancer, including basal cell cancer and squamous cell cancer, appear to have increased incidence for common biologics used for psoriasis and psoriatic arthritis, especially with previous exposure to PUVA. Therefore, clinicians should conduct total body skin exams at baseline and periodically [6].

Physicians, as key decision-makers in the treatment process, face constraints that contribute to the observed prescription patterns.

9 Geographic Distribution Challenges

The geographic distribution of biologic prescriptions in dermatology reflects a complex landscape, as evidenced by the analysis of data from the Centers for Medicare and Medicaid Services Medicare Provider Utilization and Payment Data: Part D (2013–2015) [10]. Among the 11,390 dermatologists included in the study, 26.3% were identified as prescribers of injectable biologics (IB) [10]. The national density (per 100,000 people) of IB-prescribing dermatologists was 7.22 across the US. However, the study revealed substantial disparities, with only 24.8% of counties having at least one dermatologist prescribing IB [10]. Metropolitan areas exhibited varying densities, ranging from 8.07 to 8.12, while urban populations greater than 20,000 demonstrated densities of 4.55 and 6.5 in areas adjacent and nonadjacent to metropolitan regions, respectively [10]. Populations under 2,500 considered to be completely rural or urban counties demonstrated densities between 2.31 and 2.35. In rural counties, 96.4–97.6% lacked such specialists [10]. Notably, 75% of the 3131 US counties had no dermatologists prescribing IB [10]. This data highlights the challenges in geographic accessibility, emphasizing the need for strategies to address regional disparities in biologic and immunomodulator therapy for dermatological treatment.

10 Role of Biologic Coordinators in Patient Management

In order to maximize efficiency and facilitate a fluid journey for patients from prescription to drug acquisition, Biologic Coordinators entered the practice of dermatology. Any trained staff at a medical practice can serve as biologic coordinators to help navigate the complexities of patient access on behalf of those prescribing biologics. Often, they serve as an additional source of education for the drug and disease state. However, some of their most important implications for a dermatology practice includes communicating with insurance providers, completing enrollment forms, reviewing benefit verifications, submitting prior authorizations, writing appeals and letters of medical necessity, directing patient assistance and bridge programs, and coordinating all efforts of specialty pharmacies and manufacturer HUBs. These often-convoluted tasks and procedures may serve as barriers, draining resources in terms of time, resources, and patience which could contribute to the disparities in prescribing [10].

Unfortunately, various practices could face unique challenges and limitations that limit the feasibility of these coordinators. One significant challenge revolves around the cost implications for dermatological practices. For smaller practices, sustaining experienced and skilled Biologic Coordinators might not be financially feasible. Additionally, the time commitment required for effective coordination, including navigating insurance complexities, and completing administrative tasks, can be substantial. The varying levels of experience among Biologic Coordinators contribute to a learning curve, potentially affecting the speed and efficiency of patient access. Striking a balance between cost considerations, the time commitment required, and the need for experienced professionals remains a critical aspect of optimizing the role of Biologic Coordinators in dermatological practices.

However, not all practices necessitate the need for biological coordinators, and some have staff such as medical assistants doing the work, which is dependent on the volume of prescriptions from the providers. For practices with volume worthy of prescriptions, offices are often seen utilizing a dedicated biologic coordinator. Usually in a given office, there is a point person that is the liaison between prescription to medication to patient. Acknowledging these limitations is essential for implementing strategies to enhance their impact while addressing associated challenges.

11 Impact of Prior Authorizations on Patient Care

The impact of prior authorizations (PAs) on patient care is a multifaceted issue with both advantages and disadvantages. While prior authorizations were initially designed to control costs, improve quality, and ensure that patients receive evidence-based and cost-effective treatments, they actually lead to decreased access, delays in care, decreased patient satisfaction, and increased clinician burnout. The process can be time-consuming for both clinicians and administrative staff, with physicians spending an average of 14 h per week on prior authorizations [11]. Moreover, prior authorizations may not always account for unique patient circumstances or the most up-to-date research, leading to potential denials or delays in needed care. Specifically, in a retrospective review of PAs at Beth Israel Deaconess Medical Center, 8.1% of medications prescribed required prior authorization, while 55.2% of patients prescribed medications were biological agents requiring Pas [12]. In this review, it was found that pharmacy intervention resulted in shorter time to PA submission (4 days vs. 1 day) and decision (6 days vs. 1 day), as well as significantly higher approval rates (63.9% vs. 80.6%) [12].

One study conducted by Carlisle et al. quantified the substantial administrative burden and costs associated with PAs in dermatology practices. The research quantified the impact of PAs on dermatology practices, revealing that in September 2016 alone, 626 PAs were generated from 9512 patient encounters, costing a median of $6.72 per PA [13]. Notably, biologic medication PAs incurred even higher costs, with a median of $15.80 each and prolonged processing times of up to 31 business days. Despite the high costs and administrative burden, approval rates varied, with procedures having a 99.6% approval rate compared to 78.9% for biologics and 58.2% for other medications [13]. Furthermore, the study highlighted that a significant portion of initially denied PAs were subsequently approved upon appeal, underscoring the inefficiencies in the current PA system. These findings demonstrate the urgent need for PA reform in dermatology to streamline processes, reduce costs, and ultimately improve patient outcomes [13].

The burden of prior authorizations can contribute to clinician burnout, as clinicians may choose to avoid ordering necessary treatments or testing to circumvent administrative hurdles. While payers often view prior authorizations as essential for promoting healthcare value, clinicians frequently experience firsthand the challenges and delays they impose on patient care. To explore the impact of PAs on dermatological practice, the American Academy of Dermatology (AAD) conducted a survey which found that 96.5% reported PAs delaying or preventing proper treatment and more than 66% reporting that PAs negatively affect at least 1 patient daily [14]. An unfortunate finding was that some practitioners only prescribe within formularies and refused to undertake Pas [14].

This, in combination with the added administrative burden and costs that are passed onto the patient demonstrates the clear need to streamline and optimize the prior authorization process to ensure that patient care remains paramount while minimizing administrative burdens and delays in care.

12 Understanding Medication Cost: Considerations and Terminology

12.1 Formulary and Its Implications

When discussing medication accessibility, it is crucial to address the cost of medications and the factors influencing it. Insurance companies employ various algorithms to construct their formularies, dictating which medications are covered and at what cost to the patient. Typically, medications are placed into tiers within these formularies, with lower tiers indicating greater coverage by insurance and higher tiers requiring patients to bear a larger portion of the cost, often in the form of higher copays [15]. Biologic medications are often positioned at the highest tiers, which may entail increased patient responsibility depending on insurance coverage [16]. The determination of a medication's tier within a formulary hinges on the combination of several factors, including its wholesale acquisition price (WAC), duration on the market, and supporting clinical data (cost-per-responder analyses). While many biologic medications are included in formularies, their accessibility is curtailed by substantial copays, step therapy dictated by managed care and the need for prior authorizations [16]. These obstacles are handled differently based on coverage and state.

13 Advocacy and Its Role in Medication Access

Advocacy plays a pivotal role in ensuring medication accessibility through various channels, each addressing different aspects of the complex healthcare landscape. National dermatological associations, including the American Academy of Dermatology (AAD), National Eczema Association (NEA), and National Psoriasis Foundation (NPF), are instrumental in advocating for improved medication accessibility.

These associations, alongside others, are nonprofit organizations representing both dermatologists and patients. They promote evidence-based practices in legislation and regulation to ensure equitable access to dermatologic treatments. They accomplish this through lobbying, engaging in public awareness campaigns, promoting research, and collaborating with healthcare stakeholders [17–19].

Effective advocacy for medication access necessitates collaboration among stakeholders, including patient advocacy groups, healthcare providers, policymakers, and pharmaceutical companies. Transparency, accountability, and a focus on patient-centered outcomes should underpin advocacy initiatives to ensure medication access remains a priority and patients' needs are addressed adequately. By fostering dialogue and collaboration among stakeholders, advocacy efforts can drive positive change in healthcare policies and practices, ultimately enhancing medication accessibility and improving patient outcomes.

14 Specialty Pharmacies: Navigating Their Significance

Specialty pharmacies are used for rare diseases, hard to manage complexities, and expensive medications that are not available at local pharmacies. The pharmacists and staff are trained to assist patients in managing uncommon medications in comparison to common medications available at local pharmacies. Specialty pharmacies serve as indispensable resources in ensuring patient access, affordability, and effective management of specialty medications, including biologics [20]. Central to their role is the coordination of care, with a strong emphasis on patient-centeredness, specialty pharmacies facilitate seamless communication among healthcare providers, patients, and insurance companies to optimize care delivery and treatment outcomes for the patient. By serving as a central hub for medication-related inquiries and concerns, they streamline the care process and alleviate administrative burdens from healthcare providers.

One of the functions of specialty pharmacies is to assist patients in navigating the complexities of insurance coverage, reimbursement, and financial assistance programs. This includes helping patients understand their insurance benefits, accessing copay assistance programs, and facilitating enrollment in patient assistance programs (PAPs) offered by pharmaceutical manufacturers. By leveraging their expertise in insurance navigation, specialty pharmacies empower patients to overcome financial barriers and gain access to life-changing medications.

Moreover, specialty pharmacies play a pivotal role in medication adherence support, leveraging various strategies to enhance patient compliance and persistence with treatment regimens [21]. Through proactive medication counseling, refill reminders, and adherence monitoring, they help patients comply to prescribed therapies and achieve optimal treatment outcomes [21]. This comprehensive approach to medication management not only improves patient compliance but also contributes to better clinical outcomes and quality of life.

In essence, specialty pharmacies serve as invaluable partners in the healthcare ecosystem, providing tailored support and resources to patients with complex or chronic conditions. By championing patient access, affordability, and adherence to specialty medications, they play a critical role in enhancing patient care and ultimately improving health outcomes.

15 Patient Support Programs

There are multiple ways that patients prescribed financially cumbersome medications can obtain their medications. In the following section, we detail some of these avenues, including copay cards, patient assistance programs, as well as advocacy/foundation support.

16 Copay Cards: Facilitating Cost-Sharing

Copay cards play a crucial role in alleviating the financial burden associated with rising out-of-pocket (OOP) costs for prescription medications per the Centers for Medicare and Medicaid. These programs, often established by pharmaceutical manufacturers, offer patients a lifeline, especially those facing chronic diseases requiring regular medication. Patients typically become aware of copay cards through their healthcare providers or pharmacies, often when expressing concerns about the affordability of their prescribed medications. While the application process for copay cards is generally perceived as quick and straightforward, some may encounter challenges in staying updated on changes or updates to their cards, necessitating ongoing vigilance and communication with multiple stakeholders [22].

Copay cards serve as a vital resource for patients, enabling them to afford their prescribed medications and adhere to their treatment regimens. Patients report significant savings each month, reduced stress and worry about medication costs, and improved mental health due to the alleviation of financial strain. Importantly, copay cards facilitate medication adherence, a critical factor in managing chronic conditions and improving overall health outcomes. However, patients exhibit varying levels of awareness and understanding regarding copay accumulators and maximizers, which are introduced by payers to counteract the benefits of copay cards. Accumulators, which do not count copay card payments towards deductibles or OOP maximums, are generally viewed negatively by patients, as they result in increased OOP costs and potential financial strain. Maximizers, while still posing challenges, are perceived more favorably by patients as they evenly distribute copay assistance throughout the year, aiding in budgeting and planning for medication expenses.

Looking ahead, patients express apprehension and concern about potential limitations or non-availability of copay cards in the future. The prospect of losing copay card access raises significant challenges for patients, who may consider switching medications or even forgoing treatment altogether due to financial constraints. Patients emphasize the essential role of copay cards in maintaining their health and quality of life, highlighting the critical need for ongoing support and access to affordable medications. In summary, copay cards serve as a vital resource for patients, enabling them to navigate the financial complexities of accessing prescription medications, but challenges such as copay accumulators and maximizers, as well as potential limitations on copay card availability, underscore the ongoing need for patient support programs to ensure medication affordability and adherence for individuals managing chronic diseases. Additionally, with the recent appearance of biosimilar medications, a copay card may not always be available, augmenting the cost constraints.

17 Patient Assistance Programs/Advocacy Programs: Bridging Financial Gaps

Patient assistance programs (PAPs), are instrumental in facilitating access to medications, particularly for uninsured or underinsured individuals. These programs, typically established by pharmaceutical companies, aim to bridge the gap between patients and necessary treatments. PAP's are based on income and need, and the minimum amount varies from sponsor to sponsor. However, as highlighted by a literature review conducted by Felder et al. in 2011, while PAPs have demonstrated significant clinical benefits for patients, they can also introduce additional burdens for both prescribing physicians and patients due to cumbersome paperwork requirements [23].

To mitigate the burden of paperwork on prescribing physicians, it is essential to explore alternative support mechanisms. Biologic coordinators, specialty pharmacies, and patient advocacy programs offer valuable assistance in navigating the complexities of PAPs, as discussed in other sections of this paper. These resources can streamline the application process, provide guidance on documentation requirements, and facilitate communication between healthcare providers, patients, and pharmaceutical companies.

At the same time, advocacy groups are separate entities to assist with obtaining medications. These groups, such as the National Psoriasis Foundation, National Eczema Association, PAN foundation and many others may offer resources or financial assistance for navigation of the journey.

By leveraging these support systems, healthcare professionals can optimize the utilization of PAPs, ensuring that eligible patients receive timely access to essential medications without undue administrative burden.

18 Bridge Programs: Ensuring Uninterrupted Treatment

The process of getting medication can be a cumbersome process. To ensure continuation of therapy, some pharmaceutical companies or manufacturers have bridge programs in place which act to prevent coverage gaps or delays, continuation of therapy, and prevent a financial burden on patients while maneuvering coverage. Each manufacturer typically has specific requirements and usually provides these programs to commercially insured patients. Generally, the practice either needs to submit the prescription to the specialty pharmacy which handles the programs, prior authorizations, and appeals for the practice or undertake this by themselves.

19 Additional Challenges in Dermatological Treatment

19.1 Impact of Accumulators and Maximizers on Patients and Practices

Accumulator programs disallowed patients previously utilizing manufacturer-provided financial assistance, such as coupons or copay cards, from being credited towards their annual out-of-pocket obligations under their health plans. Consequently, patients would face unexpected and exorbitant costs once their manufacturer assistance is depleted or when seeking additional medications or services.

Since September 29, 2023 a federal court recently invalidated a Trump-era rule allowing insurers to exclude drug manufacturer co-pay support coupons from patients' annual cost-sharing caps, also known as copay accumulator programs [24]. Advocacy groups challenged the rule, arguing that copay support should count towards patients' cost-sharing obligations. The court sided with the plaintiffs, stating that the rule contradicted existing regulations and the Affordable Care Act's definition of "cost sharing." Although the verdict's objective is to reduce patient cost, the downstream effect of the ruling may eventually impact drug manufacturers and patients, it is currently unclear if the ruling will be appealed. In response, patient advocacy groups, such as the Immune Deficiency Foundation, have noted that they will continue to advocate for broader bans on copay accumulator programs [24].

In the same vein, maximizer programs aim to exhaust the maximum value of manufacturer assistance throughout the plan year without accounting for these amounts towards patients' annual cost-sharing limits. Whether by evenly distributing assistance monthly or front-loading payments, maximizer programs prevent patients from receiving credit towards their deductibles or out-of-pocket maximums, leading to heightened financial burdens when seeking further healthcare services or medications. The sudden realization of substantial out-of-pocket expenses can deter patients from adhering to prescribed therapies, potentially compromising their health outcomes. The lack of transparency surrounding these programs exacerbates patient confusion and frustration, as they are often blindsided by unexpected costs.

Practices are impacted by accumulator and maximizer programs as physicians share treatment goals with patients. When prescribing medication, the challenges of addressing the financial concerns and capabilities of patients should always be balanced with ensuring feasibility and access to ensure optimal treatment outcomes. Providers are prominent stakeholders in patient success, and barriers in prescribing treatment may potentially impede patient care.

In summary, accumulator and maximizer programs have profound implications for both patients and healthcare providers, undermining efforts to improve medication access and adherence while exacerbating financial strain within the healthcare system. Addressing the impact of these programs requires collaborative efforts among stakeholders, at the state and national level, to enhance transparency, mitigate financial burdens, and uphold patient-centered care principles.

20 Challenges Posed by Step Therapy

Although the intention of "step therapy" is to ensure cost effectiveness is balanced with clinical reasoning, treatment regimens and recommendations are constantly changing. In navigating treatment options for various diseases, particularly chronic conditions, the question of whether to initiate therapy with antiquated traditional drug regimens vs modern targeted injectable biologics and small molecules presents a significant challenge. Moderately to severely ill patients and their physicians advocate for utilizing biologics as a first-line approach, particularly in cases where older medications may entail adverse effects and/or limited efficacy. Diseases such as psoriasis often prompt consideration of this dilemma due to the potential toxicity associated with conventional treatments like methotrexate and cyclosporine.

The emergence of biologic therapies, including, but not limited to, dupilumab, ustekinumab, secukinumab, guselkumab, bimekizumab, rizankizumab, ixekizumab, tralokinumab has offered promising alternatives for patients with these conditions. However, concerns arise regarding the necessity for prior use of traditional therapies before biologics, as mandated by some payer policies. The efficacy of older treatments in patients with moderate to severe chronic diseases is questioned by physicians and their data, while biologics manufacturers caution against assuming interchangeability among specialty drugs. Payers emphasize the importance of evidence demonstrating the long-term safety and efficacy of biologics, alongside considerations of cost-effectiveness.

Psoriasis serves as a notable case study reflecting the complexities of treatment decisions [25]. Traditional medications like methotrexate and cyclosporine, despite their established use, are burdened with significant side effects and frequent laboratory monitoring, prompting enthusiasm among dermatologists and rheumatologists for biologic alternatives. However, payer policies often require patients to undergo multiple traditional therapies before accessing biologics, raising concerns about the appropriateness of such requirements.

The challenge intensifies with the lack of comparative data between biologics and traditional therapies, further complicating the establishment of step therapy protocols. While step therapy traditionally evolved within oral drug categories with multiple entries and therapeutic comparability, its application to biologics faces unique hurdles. Limited competition and therapeutic similarity among biologic drugs make step therapy more complex, potentially necessitating a progression from one biologic agent to another.

Another challenge seen in practice is when insurers may mandate the use of off-label medications for treatment of specific health conditions, such as methotrexate for atopic dermatitis without formal FDA approval [26]. Then, paradoxically, insurers cite off-label use as the reason for coverage denial when a healthcare provider requests a specific medication for the treatment of a specific condition.

Achieving consensus on coverage guidelines for biologics remains elusive, with differing perspectives among clinicians, payers, and policy experts. The dialogue surrounding step therapy and biologics reflects ongoing efforts to balance timely access, affordability, and clinical evidence. While challenges persist, there is optimism that evolving strategies and collaborative approaches will ultimately guide the development of consensus-based clinical guidelines, facilitating informed treatment decisions for patients with chronic conditions.

21 Navigating Buy-and-Bill Procedures

In order to supply patients with on-demand treatment, providers participate in the Buy and Bill model of reimbursement. In this way, providers purchase the treatment or drug for patients that can be stored locally, whether on site or somewhere appropriately nearby. Typically, the cost of the drugs are reimbursed by Medicare Part B [27]. Afterwards, practices work to obtain prior authorizations for treatment underway while submitting the claim, or bill, for reimbursement from the payer.

The Buy-and-Bill approach offers several advantages for healthcare practices, including enhanced control over the drug supply chain. By managing procurement, storage, and administration internally, practices can ensure the integrity and authenticity of medications. In addition, direct dispensal to patients and bypassing an outside system, including prior authorizations and a pharmacy, may bring an ease to obstacles and bureaucracy for patients. Another advantage is the possibility of another positive revenue stream for a Dermatology office or department.

Drawbacks can especially be burdensome for practices with limited resources, including staff and space. The upfront financial risk associated with purchasing medications and the need to manage extensive drug inventories can pose challenges for some practices. Additionally, resource constraints, including time and staffing limitations, may hinder the effective implementation of Buy-and-Bill practices, prompting some organizations to explore alternative delivery models.

For practices considering the transition to Buy-and-Bill, careful planning and preparation are essential. Key priorities include securing insurance approvals for specific treatments, ensuring an adequate number of licensed clinicians for administration, and implementing robust inventory management systems. Training staff and optimizing workflows can help streamline the Buy-and-Bill process, ultimately improving patient care and practice efficiency.

22 Conclusion

22.1 Summary of Key Findings

The advent of small molecule and biologic medications has sparked a revolution in medical care, transforming not only dermatology but various fields of medicine. With superior efficacy and a reduced side effect profile compared to conventional medications like corticosteroids, these advanced therapies have ushered in a new era of treatment. However, despite their remarkable benefits, patient access remains a challenge, primarily due to cost and resource constraints. Geographical disparities, particularly evident between metropolitan and rural areas, further exacerbate this issue, highlighting the critical need for enhanced resources and support for patients in underserved regions. Addressing barriers to accessibility necessitates concerted efforts from healthcare providers, including the allocation of clinical staff and collaboration with specialty pharmacies. Advocacy initiatives play a pivotal role in mitigating these challenges, with pharmaceutical companies advocating for policy changes and offering patient financial assistance programs to alleviate financial burdens. By working together to address these barriers, stakeholders can enhance patient access to life-changing medications and improve health outcomes across a diverse population.

23 Bridge Between Theory and Practice

To improve accessibility of biologic and small molecule medications, it is important for not only the prescribing physician to be knowledgeable and comfortable with the specialized medication, but to be aware of all the topics reviewed in this chapter. Dermatologists need to stay current with the latest research and guidelines regarding the use of biologics and small molecule drugs, including indications, dosing regimens, monitoring protocols, and safety considerations. Continuing medical education and training programs play a crucial role in equipping dermatologists with the necessary skills and confidence to incorporate biologic and small molecule therapies into their clinical practice.

While having a dedicated biologic coordinator is invaluable, it may not always be feasible, particularly for smaller or rural clinics facing financial constraints. Nevertheless, the absence of in-office support staff need not be a deterrent, as specialized pharmacies offer trained personnel who can assist in coordinating patient care. Moreover, all of the players in the pursuit for access, including but not limited to the office staff, provider, specialty pharmacy, pharmaceutical company and their field reimbursement specialists often play a pivotal role in guiding patients through the process, especially in navigating the most appropriate and beneficial financial assistance program for each patient.

As the majority of injectable biologics and small molecules are newer medications, there are many limitations for prescribing them, regardless of their superior efficacy and safety profiles in comparison to previous gold standard medications. A major contributing factor to this is the cost. Due to the high cost of these specialized medications, insurance companies create barriers such as prior authorizations and step therapy. Dermatologists often encounter challenges in advocating for their patients' needs and navigating step therapy requirements, highlighting the need for greater flexibility and individualized treatment approaches. Advocacy is necessary in order to reduce these barriers and ensure that patients receive the specialized, individualized treatment for optimal outcomes.

The limitations imposed by access barriers can impede the delivery of optimal medical care in dermatology. Delayed access to biologic and small molecule therapies may result in prolonged disease activity, exacerbation of symptoms, and decreased quality of life for patients. Dermatologists face ethical dilemmas in balancing patient needs with insurance requirements, underscoring the importance of advocacy efforts to promote evidence-based and patient-centered care.

Bridging the gap between theory and practice in the use of biologic and small molecule therapies in dermatology requires a multifaceted approach that addresses physician education, coordination of care, access barriers, and advocacy efforts. By enhancing physician knowledge and comfort level, optimizing the role of biologic coordinators, advocating for patient needs, and challenging restrictive insurance practices, stakeholders can work together to ensure that patients receive timely access to the most effective treatments, ultimately improving outcomes and quality of life in dermatologic care.

24 Future Implications and Areas for Further Research

Biologic and small molecule therapies represent the forefront of medical advancement, offering targeted therapy with enhanced efficacy and a reduced side effect profile. As the availability of targeted medications continues to expand and advocacy efforts for access to these treatments intensify, we anticipate improved accessibility for patients in need of specialized therapy. However, significant geographical disparities persist across the country, presenting barriers to access. By focusing on greater education and improved navigation of the approval process, we aim to mitigate these barriers and ensure that more patients can access the specialized care they require. Through continued research and advocacy, we strive to optimize patient outcomes and advance the field of dermatological medicine.

References

1. Costello C, Maarouf M, Shi V. Navigating targeted therapeutics in dermatology: biologics and small molecules. J Drugs Dermatol. 2018;17(12):1330–1332. PMID: 30586268.
2. Kim H, Alten R, Avedano L, Dignass A, Gomollón F, Greveson K, Halfvarson J, Irving PM, Jahnsen J, Lakatos PL, Lee J, Makri S, Parker B, Peyrin-Biroulet L, Schreiber S, Simoens S, Westhovens R, Danese S, Jeong JH. The future of biosimilars: maximizing benefits across immune-mediated inflammatory diseases. Drugs. 2020;80(2):99–113. https://doi.org/10.1007/s40265-020-01256-5.Erratum.In:Drugs.2020Jul;80(10):1039-1040.PMID:32002851;PMCID:PMC7007415.
3. Leonardi CL, See K, Burge R, Sun Z, Zhang Y, Mallbris L, Garrelts A, Warren RB. Number needed to treat network meta-analysis to compare biologic drugs for moderate-to-severe psoriasis. Adv Ther. 202239(5):2256–2269. https://doi.org/10.1007/s12325-022-02065-w. Epub 2022 Mar 22. PMID: 35316500; PMCID: PMC9056462.
4. Lewitt GM. Navigating the Approval Process for Systemic Medications in Dermatology. Poster presented at: WC Hawaii; Jan 2024; Honolulu, HI.
5. Noe MH, Shin DB, Doshi JA, Margolis DJ, Gelfand JM. Prescribing patterns associated with biologic therapies for psoriasis from a United States medical records database. J Drugs Dermatol. 2019;18(8):745–750. PMID: 31424706; PMCID: PMC6764093.
6. Ortleb M, Levitt JO. Practical use of biologic therapy in dermatology: some considerations and checklists. Dermatol Online J. 2012;18(2):2 PMID: 22398223.
7. Krzysztofik M, Brzewski P, Cuber P, Kacprzyk A, Kulbat A, Richter K, Wojewoda T, Wysocki WM. Risk of melanoma and non-melanoma skin cancer in patients with psoriasis and psoriatic

arthritis treated with targeted therapies: a systematic review and meta-analysis. Pharmaceuticals (Basel). 2023;17(1):14. https://doi.org/10.3390/ph17010014.PMID:38276003;PMCID: PMC10820691.
8. Polesie S, Gillstedt M, Schmidt SAJ, et al. Use of methotrexate and risk of skin cancer: a nationwide case–control study. Br J Cancer. 2023;128:1311–9.
9. Santana AL, Felsen D, Carucci JA. Interleukin-22 and cyclosporine in aggressive cutaneous squamous cell carcinoma. Dermatol Clin. 2017;35(1):73–84. https://doi.org/10.1016/j.det.2016.07.003.PMID:27890239;PMCID:PMC5409835.
10. Feng H, Cohen JM, Neimann AL. Access to injectable biologic medications by medicare beneficiaries: geographic distribution of US dermatologist prescribers. J Dermatolog Treat. 2019;30(3):237–9. https://doi.org/10.1080/09546634.2018.1508819. Epub 2018 Sep 12 PMID: 30078341.
11. Busis NA, Khokhar B, Callaghan BC. Streamlining prior authorization to improve Care. JAMA Neurol. 2024;81(1):5–6. https://doi.org/10.1001/jamaneurol.2023.4324.
12. Popatia S, Flood KS, Golbari NM, Patel PV, Olbricht SM, Kimball AB, Porter ML. Examining the prior authorization process, patient outcomes, and the impact of a pharmacy intervention: a single-center review. J Am Acad Dermatol. 2019;81(6):1308–18.
13. Carlisle RP, Flint ND, Hopkins ZH, Eliason MJ, Duffin KC, Secrest AM. Administrative Burden and costs of prior authorizations in a dermatology department. JAMA Dermatol. 2020;156(10):1074–8.
14. Secrest AM, Asgari MM, Kourosh AS, Barbieri JS, Albrecht J. American Academy of dermatology drug pricing and transparency task force. Prior authorizations for dermatologic medications: an American Academy of Dermatology survey of US dermatology providers and staff. J Am Acad Dermatol. 2017;77(4):784–786. https://doi.org/10.1016/j.jaad.2017.05.008. PMID: 28917469
15. What Medicare Part D drug plans cover | Medicare. Medicare.gov. Published 2019. https://www.medicare.gov/drug-coverage-part-d/what-medicare-part-d-drug-plans-cover.
16. Liang SY, Haas JS, Phillips KA. Medicare formulary coverage for top-selling biologics. Nat Biotechnol. 2009;27(12):1082–4. https://doi.org/10.1038/nbt1209-1082.PMID:20010576; PMCID:PMC2845541.
17. Academy advocacy priorities. https://www.aad.org/member/advocacy/priorities
18. National Eczema Association Advocacy and Policy Priorities. National Eczema Association. https://nationaleczema.org/advocacy/
19. NPF Advocacy. www.psoriasis.org. Accessed 8 Apr 2024. https://www.psoriasis.org/advocacy/.
20. Zuckerman AD, Whelchel K, Kozlicki M, Simonyan AR, Donovan JL, Gazda NP, Mourani J, Smith AM, Young L, Ortega M, Kelley TN. Health-system specialty pharmacy role and outcomes: a review of current literature. Am J Health Syst Pharm. 2022;79(21):1906–18. https://doi.org/10.1093/ajhp/zxac212.
21. St. James GJ, Duckworth DL, Bochenek SH, Rhudy C, Zeltner M, Tagavi AB, Platt TL. Effect on medication adherence of applying a specialty pharmacy care model to nonspecialty medications: a quasi-experimental cohort study. Am J Health Syst Pharm. 2023;80(Supplement_4):S135-S142. https://doi.org/10.1093/ajhp/zxad040.
22. Cavalier D, Doherty B, Geonnotti G, Patel A, Peters W, Zona S, Shea L. Patient perceptions of Copay card utilization and policies. J Market Access Health Policy. 2023;11(1):2254586. https://doi.org/10.1080/20016689.2023.2254586.
23. Felder TM, Palmer NR, Lal LS, Mullen PD. What is the evidence for pharmaceutical patient assistance programs? A systematic review. J Health Care Poor Underserved. 2011;22(1):24–49. https://doi.org/10.1353/hpu.2011.0003.PMID:21317504;PMCID:PMC3065996.
24. Federal Court Strikes Down Copay Accumulator Programs | Insights & Resources | Goodwin Procter. www.goodwinlaw.com. https://www.goodwinlaw.com/en/insights/blogs/2023/10/federal-court-strikes-down-copay-accumulator-programs
25. Hagland M. Step therapy and biologics: no easy answers. Biotechnol Healthc. 2006;3(6):32–40. PMID: 23393486; PMCID: PMC3564371.

26. Ratchataswan T, Banzon TM, Thyssen JP, Weidinger S, Guttman-Yassky E, Phipatanakul W. Biologics for treatment of atopic dermatitis: current status and future prospect. J Allergy Clin Immunol Pract. 2021;9(3):1053–65. https://doi.org/10.1016/j.jaip.2020.11.034.PMID: 33685604;PMCID:PMC7951162.
27. Medicare Part B. Published online August 10, 2017. https://doi.org/10.1377/hpb20171008.000171

Conclusions

Neal Bhatia

Abstract The opportunities for the incorporation of systemic immunomodulators advanced significantly over the period of 2021–2023 with the release of janus kinase inhibitors and interleukin-13 inhibitors to the dermatology world for multiple indications. However, the future of other agents once thought to be prominent have since gained usage in other specialties outside of dermatology. This chapter will summarize the latest developments in new approvals of immunomodulators in dermatology as well as forecast the potential for other medications that will be introduced in 2023 and the near future.

Keywords Interleukin · Lebrikizumab · Tezepelumab · Kinase · Etrasimod · Fumaric acid · Inhibitor

The future of immunomodulation in dermatology is constantly evolving. There is a rich pipeline of biologic and systemic therapies dedicated to diseases that were once frustrating to control based on poor efficacy or safety data. Many of these agents in trials will be looking to be launched in the next several years.

1 Lebrikizumab

Lebrikizumab selectively prevents formation of the IL-13Rα1/IL-4Rα receptor signaling complex and blocking IL-13 signaling, and additionally does not prevent the binding of IL-13 to the IL-13Rα2 (decoy) receptor. As a result, these mechanisms allow cellular uptake of IL-13 [1].

In the phase 2 dose ranging trials where Lebrikizumab 125 mg was studied versus 250 mg, the 250 mg dose proved to have rapid onset and safety which prompted this dose to be evaluated in the phase 3 trials (Advocate 1 and 2). The dosage regimen

N. Bhatia (✉)
Therapeutics Clinical Research, San Diego, CA, USA
e-mail: bhatiaharbor@gmail.com

N. Bhatia (ed.), *Immunomodulators and Biologics in Dermatologic Treatment*,
https://doi.org/10.1007/978-3-031-66590-5_13

included a loading dose of 500 mg at baseline and week 2 then maintenance with 250 mg injections. The investigators concluded that Lebrikizumab 250 mg demonstrated rapid onset of action while the safety profile was consistent with previous Lebrikizumab AD studies. Most TEAEs were mild or moderate with no reported treatment discontinuation. In ADvocate 1, nearly 60% of the patients treated with Lebrikizumab achieved clinically significant improvement in EASI75 [2].

2 Tezepelumab—Anti-TSLP Ab

Tezepelumab is a monoclonal antibody that targets thymic stromal lymphopoeitin (TSLP) which mediates signaling between epithelial cells and innate immune cells to drive the pathogenesis of atopic dermatitis and potentially impact the atopic march [3]. As shown in other models, epithelial cells use TSLP to directly communicate to cutaneous sensory neurons to promote itch via the ORAI1/NFAT calcium signaling pathway as an essential regulator of TSLP release from keratinocytes. Consequently, TSLP acts directly on a subset of TRPA1-positive sensory neurons to trigger itch via calcium-dependent release which activates both primary afferent neurons and inflammatory responses in the skin and airways. In the PATHWAY trial for asthma there were few reported adverse events. However, in the atopic dermatitis trials the efficacy assessments revealed no significant separation from placebo until week 16, in addition to no significant EASI-50 even with topical steroids. A new trial with a dosage of 280 mg SQ q 2 weeks in phase 2 may be evaluated [4].

3 Amlitelimab—Anti-OX 40 Antibody

Amlitelimab is also a monoclonal antibody that targets OX40, and by inhibiting OX40 signaling by binding to antigen presenting cells' OX40 ligand there is a suppression of T-effector cells while promoting maintenance of anti-inflammatory T-regulatory cells. This interaction also targets upstream mechanisms by blocking TH1/2/17/22 paths. In the phase 2 studies for AD there were 68% of amlitelimab patients graded with their vIGA of either 0 or 1 up to Week 36, which was 24 weeks following their final dose. No hypersensitivity or other safety signals. However, one potential limiting step for dermatologists is the delivery as it is administered currently as an IV dose Q4W until Week 12 with a loading dose at baseline, so the development of a subcutaneous delivery will open more opportunities in dermatology [5].

4 Bruton Tyrosine Kinases

Signaling via the Bruton Tyrosine Kinase pathway is connected to a number of upstream and downstream proteins/receptors, although the distinction is that it functions as a non-receptor mediator tyrosine kinase. One of the principal functions is to connect with toll-like receptor (TLR) signaling as well as downstream transcription factors and protein kinases in dendritic cells and neutrophils. Consequently, this influences induction of p-BTK expression along with concomitant increase in IL-23, and TNF-α in $CD11c^{+}$ dendritic cells [6]. Rilzabrutinib represents one of the earliest Bruton Tyrosine Kinase Inhibitors (BTKi) with highly selective covalent binding and auto Ab-mediated FcgR signaling. This inhibits IgE-mediated, Fc«R-dependent immune mechanisms in human basophils and mast cells. Currently it is being studied in trials for atopic dermatitis and pemphigus vulgaris [7].

5 Ritlecitinib: TEC Non-receptor Kinases

Pending the launch in mid to late 2023 for alopecia areata and in early phase trials for vitiligo, Ritlecitinib will come to market as the first of the JAK 3/TEC Kinases which function as a non-receptor kinase [8–11]. It is currently being studied at various doses between 10, 30, and 50 mg for each of the indications with or without a 200 mg loading dose.

A phase 2b–3 trial was conducted at 118 sites in 18 countries involving 718 enrolled subjects 12 years of age and older with and alopecia areata involving 50% or greater scalp surface area. The subjects were randomized to either oral ritlecitinib or placebo once-daily for 24 weeks, with or without a 4-week loading dose (50, 30, 10, 200 mg loading dose followed by 50, or 200 mg loading dose followed by 30 mg), followed by a 24-week extension period. The primary endpoint was Severity of Alopecia Tool (SALT) score 20 or less at week 24 assessed in all assigned patients independent of whether they received treatment. At week 24, 38 (31%) of 124 patients in the ritlecitinib 200 + 50 mg group, 27 (22%) of 121 patients in the 200 + 30 mg group, 29 (23%) of 124 patients in the 50 mg group, 17 (14%) of 119 patients in the 30 mg group, and two (2%) of 130 patients in the placebo group had a response based on SALT score 20 or less. The difference in response rate based on SALT score 20 or less between the placebo and the ritlecitinib 200 + 50 mg group was 29.1% (95% CI 21.2–37.9; $p < 0.0001$), 20.8% (13.7–29.2; $p < 0.0001$) for the 200 + 30 mg group, 21.9% (14.7–30.2; $p < 0.0001$) for the 50 mg group, and 12.8% (6.7–20.4; $p = 0.0002$) for the 30 mg group. Up to week 48 and including the follow-up period, AEs had been reported in 108 (82%) of 131 patients in the ritlecitinib 200 + 50 mg group, 105 (81%) of 129 patients in the 200 + 30 mg group, 110 (85%) of 130 patients in the 50 mg group, 106 (80%) of 132 patients in the 30 mg group, 47 (76%) of 62 patients in the 10 mg group, 54 (83%) of 65 patients placebo to ritlecitinib 200 +

50 mg in the extension period, and 57 (86%) of 66 patients in the placebo to 50 mg group [12].

6 Tyrosine Kinase 2 Inhibitors

Selective inhibition of the tyrosine kinase 2 enzymatic pathways results in the blockade of production of IL-17 by lymphocytes from the stimulus of IL-23. Specifically, tyrosine kinase 2 (TYK 2) mediates signaling of Type I cytokines (IL-23, IL-12, and interferons) involved in psoriasis pathogenesis. Deucravacitinib is a novel oral agent that selectively inhibits TYK2 which uniquely binds to the regulatory domain, as opposed to the catalytic domain representing the ATP binding sites. The allosteric inhibition of TYK2 has proven to be nearly 100 times more selective than binding either JAK 1 or JAK 3, and nearly 2000 times more selective than binding for JAK 2 in assays [13].

Unlike the three Janus Kinase enzymes, Tyrosine Kinase 2 has primarily immune mediated effects without metabolic effects such as hematopoiesis, lipid metabolism, and bone metabolism. More specifically, when paired with a JAK enzyme, TYK2 mediates the activity of the receptor binding of IL-12, IL-23, and type I interferons. By contrast, JAK2 impacts the metabolism and receptor binding of erythropoietin, leptin, growth hormone, GM-CSF, and thrombopoeitin in addition to the mechanisms of the other JAK enzymes [14–17].

The POETYK trials have been widely published for introducing deucravacitinib to the market for another oral option for psoriasis, as many dermatologists have been abandoning methotrexate and cyclosporine due to safety and immunosuppression risks as well as apremilast for concerns of efficacy. The data from these trials (POETYK PSO-1, PSO-2, and LTE trials $n = 1519$) demonstrated favorable efficacy at 6 mg daily compared to both placebo and apremilast as well as safe and effective control of psoriasis in the long-term extension trials. There were no trends or clinically meaningful changes in multiple hematologic, lipid, and chemistry parameters and signature lab changes associated with JAK 1/2/3 inhibitors were not observed over 2 years of deucravacitinib exposure. There were rare CTCAE grade ≥ 3 laboratory abnormalities and treatment discontinuations over the first 52 weeks [18–20].

Deucravacitinib has also shown to be an effective agent for the treatment of systemic lupus erythematosus. In the Deucravacitinib Ph2 PAISLEY trial for SLE, the rationale for TYK2 Inhibition was to bind and inactivate the TYK2 regulatory domain with the safety based on the lack of impact on metabolic or hematopoietic pathways. Similar to psoriasis and psoriatic arthritis, the pairings of TYK2 with JAK 1 or 2 inhibit IL-12, IL-23, and Interferons with the observation of inhibiting Anti-Sm and Anti-DS DNA antibody activity [21]. Patients enrolled in the trial were seropositive for these antibodies but did not have any visceral consequences from lupus and otherwise met SLICC criteria. They were randomized to either placebo or Deucravacitinib at 3 mg bid, 6 mg bid, or 12 mg once daily with a gradual steroid taper and assessment at 32 weeks. Another steroid taper was performed prior to the final assessment at 48 weeks. The improvements in the Systemic Lupus Erythematosus Responder Index at the 3 mg bid dose were the most impressive reaching nearly 58.2% which was superior to those observed in the other dosage arms. There were similar superiority findings at the same dose with the CLASI-50 score assessments and the Joint Count 50 [21].

The inhibition of tyrosine kinase 2 will continue to not only be a target for new molecules but also for combination approaches given the safety profiles. Of note TAK-279 Tyrosine Kinase 2 Inhibitor is currently in Phase 2b clinical trial for psoriasis with PASI endpoints 5, 15 and 30 mg versus placebo at 12 weeks. Early trials have reported that 46% of pts achieved PASI 90 and 33% achieved PASI 100. Phase 3 trials are starting in 2023 for PsO, soon for PsA, SLE, and inflammatory bowel disease [22].

7 SAR441566: An Oral TNF Inhibitor?

Unlike biologic TNF antagonists, there is preserved signaling through TNFR2 which might decrease infectious risks associated with biologic TNF inhibitors if delivered through an oral pathway. A molecule under investigation known as SAR441566 binds to a pocket in the center of the soluble TNFα trimer to induce allosteric stabilization of a transient intermediate form. However, this asymmetric trimer cannot bind TNFR1 as well and therefore TNFR1 signaling is impaired. Currently there are trials underway in dermatology and rheumatology to determine efficacy and safety [23].

8 Fumaric Acid and Etrasimod: Will They Come Back to Dermatology?

The mechanism of action of Fumaric acid was thought to be through multiple immunomodulating and anti-oxidative properties. Fumaric Acid is known to start as a prodrug Dimethyl Fumarate (DMF), and after hydrolysis becomes active with pleiotropic immunomodulating properties inhibiting the actions mediated by Th17- and Th1 as seen in patients with psoriasis [24].

For many years fumaric acid was evaluated in trials for psoriasis and psoriatic arthritis, but as monotherapy was not clearly established in a routine. In addition, most trials that were conducted in Europe were not replicated for approval in the US market. One European study and publication reviewed the efficacy and safety of fumaric acid esters (FAEs) as monotherapy and in combination with phototherapy or methotrexate in patients with psoriasis treated in Germany. This was a single center report involving 859 patients of which 626 received FAE monotherapy while 123 received FAEs with concomitant phototherapy and 110 received FAEs with methotrexate. A median duration of 1 year was observed in all three treatment subcohorts ($P = 0.70$) from initiation of FAE treatment to a 50% response rate. A 50% response rate for PASI 75 was achieved in the FAE monotherapy subcohort after a median of 3 years of treatment, in the FAEs + phototherapy subcohort after 6.7 years and in the FAEs + methotrexate subcohort after 8.1 years ($P = 0.001$). In the study, 49.0% reported adverse events, most of which were GI related, while only 2.3% of patients reported serious adverse events. More importantly, these patients were safely studied for this extended duration [25].

Over the past few years Fumaric Acid has been studied against multiple IL-17 and IL-23 inhibitors including secukinumab and guselkumab. The PRIME trial involved a comparison of fumaric acid vs secukinamab in 200 patients. At week 24, significantly more patients receiving secukinumab compared with FAEs achieved PASI 75 response (89.5% vs. 33.7%, $P < 0.001$), and PASI 90 response (75.2% vs. 18.9%, $P < 0.001$) while most discontinuations were mostly due to adverse events, and occurred more frequently in the FAE group (1.9% vs. 40.0%) [26].

The CHANGE trial was a phase III open-label study with blinded assessment of efficacy conducted in Germany. The subjects were randomized 1:1 to either risankizumab 150 mg SQ at weeks 0, 4 and 16 or oral FAEs at increasing doses from 30 mg daily (week 0) up to 720 mg daily (weeks 8–24). Key efficacy endpoints were met at week 24 for risankizumab ($n = 60$) versus FAEs ($n = 60$) ($P < 0.001$) with PASI-90 as the primary endpoint (83.3% vs. 10.0%), the rates of gastrointestinal disorders, flushing, lymphopenia and headache were higher in the FAE group. One patient receiving risankizumab reported a serious infection (influenza, which required hospitalization). There were no malignancies, tuberculosis or opportunistic infections in either treatment arm [27].

Etrasimod is a Sphingosine 1-Phosphate Receptor Modulator which was previously studied in phase 2 in atopic dermatitis and has been in phase 3 for ulcerative colitis. In the ADVISE trial, where the primary outcome was percent change in EASI score from baseline at week 12, 140 subjects were randomized to etrasimod 2 mg ($n = 47$), 1 mg ($n = 47$) or placebo ($n = 46$). At Week 12, percent change in EASI score was 57.2% in the 2 mg etrasimod group compared to 48.4% in the placebo group ($p = 0.18$). A significantly greater proportion of participants receiving etrasimod 2 mg achieved vIGA-AD scores of 0 or 1 with a $\geq$ 2-point improvement at Week 12 versus placebo but EASI-75 response was not statistically significant versus placebo. Treatment-emergent AEs occurred in 59.6%, 40.4% and 47.8% of participants receiving etrasimod 2 mg, 1 mg and placebo, respectively and there were no serious AEs or deaths [28]. Since this trial did not result in endpoint success, subsequent investigations involving etrasimod have not been directed to treatment of dermatology conditions and are mainly focused on gastrointestinal disorders.

9 Conclusions

As summarized in these chapters as well as in the updates of clinical research in dermatology, the potential applications for immunomodulators continue to expand but the understanding of their mechanisms and safety profiles need to be further elucidated to practitioners. The understanding and subsequent utility of topical, systemic, and biologic immunomodulators to change patient outcomes, and to alter the progression of diseases rather than just serve to suppress inflammation. As more clinical trials with immunomodulators expand to be considered for dermatological conditions, more potential options will be available to patients with diseases that were missing therapies that impacted their processes to bring long-term safe improvements not only in their skin but their overall health and quality of life.

References

1. Simpson EL, et al. Efficacy and safety of lebrikizumab (an anti-IL-13 monoclonal antibody) in adults with moderate-to-severe atopic dermatitis inadequately controlled by topical corticosteroids: a randomized, placebo-controlled phase II trial (TREBLE). J Am Acad Dermatol. 2018;78:863–871.e11.
2. Silverberg JL, et al. Two phase 3 trials of lebrikizumab for moderate-to-severe atopic dermatitis. N Engl J Med. 2023;388:1080–109.
3. Wilson S, Bautista D, et al. The epithelial cell-derived atopic dermatitis cytokine TSLP activates neurons to induce itch. Cell 2013;155:285–95.
4. Simpson E, et al. Tezepelumab, an antiethymic stromal lymphopoietin monoclonal antibody, in the treatment of moderate to severe atopic dermatitis: a randomized phase 2a clinical trial. J Am Acad Dermatol Eric. https://doi.org/10.1016/j.jaad.2018.11.059
5. Webb GJ, et al. OX40, OX40L and autoimmunity: a comprehensive review. Clin Rev Allergy Immunol. 2016;50:312–22
6. Nadeem A, Ahmad SF, Al-Harbi NO, et al. Bruton's tyrosine kinase inhibitor suppresses imiquimod-induced psoriasis-like inflammation in mice through regulation of IL-23/IL-17A in innate immune cells. Int Immunopharmacol. 2020;80: 106215. https://doi.org/10.1016/j.intimp.2020.106215.
7. Langrish C, et al. Preclinical efficacy and anti-inflammatory mechanisms of action of the Bruton tyrosine kinase inhibitor Rilzabrutinib for immune-mediated disease. J Immunol. 2021;206:1454–68.
8. Perera E, et al. Alopecia areata. Curr Probl Dermatol. 2015;47:67–75.
9. Park H, Yu DA, Kwon O. Janus kinase inhibitors: an innovative treatment for alopecia areata. J Dermatol. 2019;46(8):724–30.
10. Smith SE, Neier SC, Reed BK, Davis TR, Sinnwell JP, Eckel-Passow JE, Sciallis GF, Wieland CN, Torgerson RR, Gil D, Neuhauser C, Schrum AG, Multiplex matrix network analysis of protein complexes in the human TCR signalosome. Sci Signal. 2016;9(439):rs7.
11. King B, Guttman-Yassky E, Peeva E, et al. A phase 2a randomized, placebo-controlled study to evaluate the efficacy and safety of the oral Janus kinase inhibitors ritlecitinib and brepocitinib in alopecia areata: 24-week results. J Am Acad Dermatol. 2021;85(2):379–87.
12. King B, et al. Efficacy and safety of ritlecitinib in adults and adolescents with alopecia areata: a randomized, double-blind, multicenter, phase 2b–3 trial. Lancet. 2023;401(10387):1518–29.
13. Burke JR, Cheng L, Gillooly KM, et al. Autoimmune pathways in mice and humans are blocked by pharmacological stabilization of the TYK2 pseudokinase domain. Sci Transl Med. 2019;11(502):eaaw1736.

14. Banerjee S, Biehl A, Gadina M, Hasni S, Schwartz DM. JAK-STAT signaling as a target for inflammatory and autoimmune diseases: current and future prospects. Drugs. 2017;77(8):939.
15. Xie J, LeBaron MJ, Nevalainen MT, Rui H. Role of tyrosine kinase Jak2 in prolactin-induced differentiation and growth of mammary epithelial cells. J Biol Chem. 2002;277:14020–30
16. Jiang L, Li Z, Rui L. Leptin stimulates both JAK2-dependent and JAK2-independent signaling pathways. J Biol Chem. 2008;283(42):28066–73.
17. Burke JR, Cheng L, Gillooly KM, et al. Autoimmune pathways in mice and humans are blocked by pharmacological stabilization of the TYK2 pseudokinase domain. Sci Transl Med. 2019;11(502):eaaw1736. https://doi.org/10.1126/scitranslmed.aaw1736
18. Papp K, Gordon K, Thaçi D, et al. Phase 2 trial of selective tyrosine kinase 2 inhibition in psoriasis. N Engl J Med. 2018;379(14):1313–21. https://doi.org/10.1056/NEJMoa1806382.
19. Winthrop KL. The emerging safety profile of JAK inhibitors in rheumatic disease. Nat Rev Rheumatol. 2017;13(4):234–43.
20. Armstrong AW, Gooderham M, Warren RB, et al. Deucravacitinib versus placebo and apremilast in moderate to severe plaque psoriasis: efficacy and safety results from the 52-week, randomized, double-blinded, placebo-controlled phase 3 POETYK PSO-1 trial. J Am Acad Dermatol. 2023;88(1):29–39. https://doi.org/10.1016/j.jaad.2022.07.002.
21. Morand E, Pike M, Merrill JT, et al. Deucravacitinib, a tyrosine kinase 2 inhibitor, in systemic lupus erythematosus: a phase II, randomized, double-blind, placebo-controlled trial. Arthritis Rheumatol. 2023;75(2):242–52. https://doi.org/10.1002/art.42391.
22. https://www.healio.com/news/dermatology/20230318/takedas-tyk2-inhibitor-shows-promising-phase-2-results-in-psoriasis
23. Vugler A, O'Connell J, Nguyen MA, et al. An orally available small molecule that targets soluble TNF to deliver anti-TNF biologic-like efficacy in rheumatoid arthritis. Front Pharmacol. 2022;13:1037983. Published 2022 Nov 16. https://doi.org/10.3389/fphar.2022.1037983
24. Mrowietz U, Morrison PJ, Suhrkamp I, et al. The pharmacokinetics of fumaric acid esters reveal their in vivo effects. Trends Pharmacol Sci. 2018;39:1–12.
25. Dickel H, Bruckner T, Altmeyer P. Long-term real-life safety profile and effectiveness of fumaric acid esters in psoriasis patients: a single-centre, retrospective, observational study. J Euro Acta Dermatol Venearol. 2018;32(10):1710–27.
26. Sticherling M, Mrowietz U, Augustin M, et al. Secukinumab is superior to fumaric acid esters in treating patients with moderate-to-severe plaque psoriasis who are naive to systemic treatments: results from the randomized controlled PRIME trial. Br J Dermatol. 2017;177(4):1024–32. [Published correction appears in Br J Dermatol. 2017;177(6):1772]. https://doi.org/10.1111/bjd.15707
27. Thaçi D, Eyerich K, Pinter A, et al. Direct comparison of risankizumab and fumaric acid esters in systemic therapy-naïve patients with moderate-to-severe plaque psoriasis: a randomized controlled trial. Br J Dermatol. 2022;186(1):30–9. https://doi.org/10.1111/bjd.20481.
28. Silverberg JI, Bissonnette R, Kircik L, et al. Efficacy and safety of etrasimod, a sphingosine 1-phosphate receptor modulator, in adults with moderate-to-severe atopic dermatitis (ADVISE). J Eur Acad Dermatol Venereol. 2023;37(7):1366–74. https://doi.org/10.1111/jdv.18914.

Index

N. Bhatia (ed.), *Immunomodulators and Biologics in Dermatologic Treatment*,
https://doi.org/10.1007/978-3-031-66590-5

GPSR Compliance

The European Union's (EU) General Product Safety Regulation (GPSR) is a set of rules that requires consumer products to be safe and our obligations to ensure this.

If you have any concerns about our products, you can contact us on ProductSafety@springernature.com

In case Publisher is established outside the EU, the EU authorized representative is:

Springer Nature Customer Service Center GmbH
Europaplatz 3
69115 Heidelberg, Germany

Batch number: 10703869

Printed by Printforce, the Netherlands